The World Health Organization is a specialized agency of the United Nations with primary responsibility for international health matters and public health. Through this organization, which was created in 1948, the health professions of some 165 countries exchange their knowledge and experience with the aim of making possible the attainment by all citizens of the world by the year 2000 of a level of health that will permit them to lead a socially and economically productive life.

By means of direct technical cooperation with its Member States, and by stimulating such cooperation among them, WHO promotes the development of comprehensive health services, the prevention and control of diseases, the improvement of environmental conditions, the development of health manpower, the coordination and development of biomedical and health services research, and the planning and implementation of health programmes.

These broad fields of endeavour encompass a wide variety of activities, such as developing systems of primary health care that reach the whole population of Member countries; promoting the health of mothers and children; combating malnutrition; controlling malaria and other communicable diseases, including tuberculosis and leprosy; having achieved the eradication of smallpox, promoting mass immunization against a number of other preventable diseases; improving mental health; providing safe water supplies; and training health personnel of all categories.

Progress towards better health throughout the world also demands international cooperation in such matters as establishing international standards for biological substances, pesticides, and pharmaceuticals; formulating environmental health criteria; recommending international nonproprietary names for drugs; administering the International Health Regulations; revising the International Classification of Diseases, Injuries, and Causes of Death; and collecting and disseminating health statistical information.

Further information on many aspects of WHO's work is presented in the Organization's publications.

AIDS Prevention and Control

AIDS
Prevention and Control

Invited presentations and papers from the

World Summit of Ministers of Health
on Programmes for AIDS Prevention

JOINTLY ORGANIZED BY THE WORLD HEALTH ORGANIZATION
AND THE UNITED KINGDOM GOVERNMENT,
QUEEN ELIZABETH II CONFERENCE CENTRE,
WESTMINSTER, LONDON, 26–28 JANUARY 1988

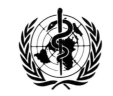

World Health Organization
Geneva

PERGAMON PRESS
OXFORD · NEW YORK · BEIJING · FRANKFURT
SÃO PAULO · SYDNEY · TOKYO · TORONTO

U.K.	Pergamon Press plc, Headington Hill Hall, Oxford OX3 0BW, England
U.S.A.	Pergamon Press Inc, Maxwell House, Fairview Park, Elmsford, New York 10523, U.S.A.
PEOPLE'S REPUBLIC OF CHINA	Pergamon Press, Room 4037, Qianmen Hotel, Beijing, People's Republic of China
FEDERAL REPUBLIC OF GERMANY	Pergamon Press GmbH, Hammerweg 6, D-6242 Kronberg, Federal Republic of Germany
BRAZIL	Pergamon Editora Ltda, Rua Eça de Queiros, 346. CEP 04011, Paraiso, São Paulo, Brazil
AUSTRALIA	Pergamon Press Australia Pty Ltd., P.O. Box 544, Potts Point, N.S.W. 2011, Australia
JAPAN	Pergamon Press, 5th Floor, Matsuoka Central Building, 1-7-1 Nishishinjuku, Shinjuku-ku, Tokyo 160, Japan
CANADA	Pergamon Press Canada Ltd., Suite No. 271, 253 College Street, Toronto, Ontario, Canada M5T 1R5

First edition 1988

Published jointly by the World Health Organization, Geneva, and Pergamon Press, Oxford.

British Library Cataloguing in Publication Data
Programmes for AIDS prevention (1988: London, England)
  AIDS Prevention and control: invited presentations and
  papers from the World Summit of Ministers of
  Health on Programmes for AIDS Prevention.
  1. Man. AIDS. Public health aspects
  I. Title II. World Health Organization
  III. Great Britain
  614.5

ISBN 92 4 156115 7 (WHO; flexicover)
ISBN 0-08-036142-0 (Pergamon; hardcover)

Typeset, printed and bound in Great Britain by
Hazell Watson & Viney Limited
Member of BPCC plc
Aylesbury, Bucks, England

Contents

v

Part V. Arming Health Workers for the AIDS Challenge

Closing Addresses

Preface

The World Summit of Ministers of Health on Programmes for AIDS Prevention held in London on 26–28 January 1988 was a striking example of international cooperation. The meeting, which was jointly organized by the Government of the United Kingdom and the World Health Organization, brought together an unprecedented number of ministers of health and representatives of United Nations agencies and intergovernmental and international nongovernmental organizations to exchange views on the role of education and information programmes in the fight against AIDS.

The London Declaration, which was adopted unanimously at the Summit, highlights the need to broaden the scope of information programmes, strengthen the exchange of information and experience among countries, and encourage throughout the world social tolerance for persons infected with HIV and with AIDS.

This volume contains: the London Declaration; the opening and closing speeches of the meeting by Her Royal Highness The Princess Royal, Mr John Moore, MP, Secretary of State for Social Services, United Kingdom, Mr Tony Newton, Minister for Health, United Kingdom, and Dr Halfdan Mahler, Director-General of the World Health Organization; the keynote speeches of Dr Jonathan Mann, Director of the WHO Global Programme on AIDS, and Sir Donald Acheson, Chief Medical Officer, Department of Health and Social Security, United Kingdom; introductions to the four technical sessions; the texts of experts' presentations; the final list of participants; and additional WHO material on AIDS.

The names of ministers, experts or delegation members whose statements made during the Summit are available are marked by an asterisk in the list of participants. Copies of those statements are available in their original format and language by writing to the Global Programme on AIDS, World Health Organization, 1211 Geneva 27, Switzerland.

We thank Mr Robert Maxwell for his collaboration in the publication of this volume.

Rt Hon. John Moore   H. Mahler, M.D.
Secretary of State   Director-General
for Social Services   World Health
United Kingdom   Organization

Opening Addresses

Her Royal Highness The Princess Royal

The Right Honourable John Moore, MP,
Secretary of State for Social Services,
United Kingdom of Great Britain and Northern Ireland

Dr Halfdan Mahler,
Director-General, World Health Organization,
Geneva, Switzerland

Her Royal Highness The Princess Royal

Your Excellencies, Ministers, Ladies and Gentlemen,

It is my pleasure to have been asked to open officially this World Summit on Programmes for AIDS Prevention. I offer a sincere welcome to all of you, ministers and delegates from so many countries, who have taken the trouble to be present here this week in London.

This Summit, as the Minister has mentioned, has been jointly organized by Her Majesty's Government and the World Health Organization. WHO's Global Programme on AIDS was launched in response to the need for a coordinated international reaction in combating the spread of the virus. One of the aims of this Summit is to consider how the Programme can best be adapted and implemented within national programmes as part of the global strategy for AIDS prevention and control.

There is a saying, which was often quoted at me in my youth, usually in relation to crime and punishment but also occasionally to personal hygiene, and one which I now quote frequently, especially in relation to health and hygiene, which is that prevention is better than cure. When there is no cure, prevention is the only answer. It is also cheaper, because the cost of AIDS in financial terms – never mind human terms – is far more than most countries can support.

It is the measures necessary for prevention and the vitally important public education which need to be highlighted and to be applied as widely and consistently as possible. We all need to learn. Ignorance in this instance is definitely not bliss.

The world community's awareness of the real risks of catching the disease can be clouded by cultural and traditional attitudes to the role of men and women and their financial state. The realities of the condition need to be explained to sufferers and carers; medically, there is still relatively little known about the origins, history, and development of the AIDS virus.

It could be said that the AIDS pandemic is a classic "own goal" scored by the human race on itself, a self-inflicted wound that only serves to remind *Homo sapiens* of his fallibility.

The real tragedy concerns the innocent victims, people who have been infected unknowingly, perhaps as the result of a blood transfusion, and the few who may have been infected knowingly by sufferers seeking revenge, but possibly, worst of all, those babies who are infected in the womb and are born with the virus. The Save the Children Fund has experience of the effects of AIDS on families in many parts of the world, including the United Kingdom.

I know these are but some aspects of a much wider problem, but they serve to illustrate the importance of the issues to be addressed at this Summit in examining how to persuade all sections of our population that AIDS presents risks not only to themselves but also to their nearest and dearest.

So far, says WHO, the global response to AIDS has been characterized by a series of delays. World summits are not quick or easy to organize and do not always produce results. Please make this one work! Make this Summit be the forerunner of the most genuine international cooperation ever seen so far! Literally millions of people could have reason to be grateful to you! Do not underestimate the long-term effects of the virus! We can put people on the moon, we can eradicate smallpox, we could stop polio; you can make a start to prevent and control AIDS!

May I wish you a very successful Summit.

The Right Honourable John Moore

SECRETARY OF STATE FOR SOCIAL SERVICES, UNITED KINGDOM
OF GREAT BRITAIN AND NORTHERN IRELAND

Your Royal Highness, Ministers, Colleagues, Ladies and Gentlemen,

I am delighted to have this opportunity to follow Her Royal Highness the Princess Royal in addressing this Summit. May I thank you, Madam, for honouring us with your presence today.

AIDS presents a growing threat to public health throughout the world, and the very large number of health ministers who are here is a measure of the seriousness of that threat. I believe that an international gathering of health ministers on this scale is completely without precedent, and I am particularly pleased that we in the United Kingdom have had the opportunity to join WHO in arranging it. May I thank you all very much for coming and wish you a very pleasant stay in London and a most constructive Summit.

The central theme of this conference is the role of public education in the fight against AIDS. Whilst in many areas in which governments become involved public education may seem something of a luxury, in this area it is an absolutely vital necessity. With no vaccine available at present to prevent HIV infection and no cure for AIDS – and with neither likely for a number of years – public education represents our best chance of reducing the dreadful toll of this disease. And I believe this to be true in the case of the population as a whole as well as of those groups, such as those who inject drugs, whose behaviour puts them at particular risk.

Over the next few days you will hear a variety of presentations dealing with information and education. Our experience here in the United Kingdom will be among them. But I would not wish to give the impression that a campaign of public education, crucial though it clearly is, will be sufficient by itself. It has to be set in the context of a general framework of action.

The United Kingdom strategy

Accordingly, we have developed a comprehensive strategy to face the challenge of AIDS. This comprises action on:

- public education
- infection control and surveillance
- research
- the development of health and other services for people with AIDS or HIV infection.

As I have said, education of the public plays the central role in our strategy. Only by influencing individual behaviour and lifestyles can we hope to contain the spread of infection. The United Kingdom Government committed £20 million to its public education campaign in November 1986, which is a reflection of the importance we attach to it. I do not want to say any more about the campaign at this stage as you will hear about our experience in considerable detail during the course of the conference.

Of the other areas of activity I have mentioned, research is obviously a major priority. We have given our Medical Research Council an additional £14.5 million over the next three years to finance a directed programme of AIDS research aimed at the development not only of vaccines against HIV but also of antiviral drugs to treat those who become infected. The Medical Research Council also receives funds for general AIDS research outside this programme. And the important pharmaceutical industry in this country is also investing heavily in this area.

As for infection control and the development of health and other services, there is a great deal going on in these fields. For example, we have adopted a number of measures to safeguard public health, such as the screening of blood donations and the heat treatment of blood products. As far as care and treatment services are concerned, we are actively seeking to develop these and to promote cooperation between our health authorities, local government, and the voluntary sector – all of which have important contributions to make. We believe there will be an increasing demand for care to be carried out in people's own homes, which will require sensitive and flexible community-based services.

General philosophy

There is a lot of work going on in the United Kingdom to tackle the challenge posed by AIDS. With the number of AIDS cases continuing to double every 10 or 11 months, such a sense of urgency is crucial. I should, however, like to emphasize three strands that form the underlying philosophy of our whole approach. These are the exercise of leadership, cooperation across the whole of society, and the importance of the international dimension.

AIDS raises many difficult cultural, ethical and practical questions. The problems are compounded by the fact that the main ways by which the infection may be transmitted involve very sensitive areas of personal behaviour. But effective action to contain and then defeat this disease is dependent on governments squarely addressing uncomfortable issues, not shying away from them. We must all give a lead to our countrymen. We must give them the facts and try to establish a general consensus on the measures to be taken. This will not be easy. It will need the exercise of political leadership and the harnessing of a general political will. But we owe it to our people to find this political will since the consequences of not doing so would be dire. I believe that the public education message has a much greater chance of general acceptance if governments give a lead and themselves demonstrate commitment to the fight against AIDS. This is why the British Government has worked so hard to produce a coordinated response across all of its departments.

The second basic strand of our approach is cooperation. Our public education campaign, for example, has not been run by the central government only; it has been very much a response from all parts of British society working together. National television and radio as well as other parts of the media have all played a major part. Education has been carried forward in schools, in prisons, in the workplace, and elsewhere. Initiatives to spread the message have been taken at local level by health and local authorities.

Voluntary bodies have also played a particularly vital role. They have delivered information rapidly and in a form most appropriate to the particular groups they assist.

The international dimension

The third strand of our approach – and it is a crucially important one – is the international dimension. As I said in the very welcome debate held in the General Assembly of the United Nations last October, AIDS is no respecter of national boundaries and we need a global response to contain it. The world must pool its knowledge on research, care, and treatment and on the effective use of information and education programmes. WHO's Global Programme on AIDS has a vitally important role here, and I am pleased that the United Kingdom Government has been able to give it substantial support. This Summit meeting is a further sign of our commitment to cooperation with WHO.

Of course, if international cooperation is to make the maximum impact it must be coordinated. It is vital to take action together. Resources are finite and we must avoid wasteful duplication. As I have said, WHO's Global Programme has a crucial role in this area. The United Kingdom has so far contributed £3.25 million to its funding. As substantial further evidence of our commitment to international action, I am very pleased to be able to announce today a large increase in that contribution. Subject to the approval of Parliament, we intend to provide £4.5 million from our Overseas Aid Programme towards the funding of the WHO Global Programme in 1988/89.

We must not forget that global action by governments and international agencies must be, and is being, complemented by that of other bodies such as voluntary organizations. I was very pleased to see that the major British aid agencies, such as Oxfam and the Save the Children Fund – of which Her Royal Highness the Princess Royal is the President – have come together to coordinate their efforts in the fight against AIDS.

To conclude, it is clear that for the moment public information and education remain our most powerful weapons in the fight against the growing challenge of AIDS. The United Kingdom is committed to meeting this challenge and to seeking the greatest possible international cooperation in doing so. We are demonstrating this by hosting this Summit. I hope you find that it provides you with new and useful information and permits a valuable exchange of ideas and views, in the spirit of cooperation against a menace with which we must all deal.

Dr Halfdan Mahler

DIRECTOR-GENERAL, WORLD HEALTH ORGANIZATION

Your Royal Highness, Ministers, Ladies and Gentlemen,

A meeting of health ministers is an event reserved for only the most important public health concerns – and we are now opening such a summit on AIDS. I wish to express my gratitude to the Government of the United Kingdom for giving us all this precious occasion to draw strength from common purpose by generously hosting this world summit.

With AIDS, the world's quota of misery, already so full, is even fuller. Yet we see, throughout the world, evidence of an energetic response to AIDS that cannot fail to inspire and bring with it hope. What is this energy? Why do those working on AIDS seem energized, electrified, in some way possessed? When I look at the quality and dedication of those working to overcome AIDS I cannot believe that such commitment should be faddish or transitory. AIDS seems to be calling forth an urgent, deep global need to help others, to help ourselves.

The World Health Organization, your World Health Organization, is constitutionally the directing and coordinating authority on international health work, and you, ministers of health, are the main actors, the spinal cord uniting the Organization as a collectivity of Member States and the governments and people of each and every Member State.

As ministers, you have a role in determining collectively the policies of WHO and in carrying them out internationally as well as nationally in your own countries. Your governments have all enthusiastically agreed to the global policy of health for all by the year 2000 and to the global strategy to give effect to it. Fortunately, the policy and strategy for health for all by the year 2000 are operational realities – fortunately for the health of the people of the world in general and fortunately because they are the key to AIDS prevention and control.

The Global Strategy for Health for All rests on four pillars:

(1) political commitment;
(2) intersectoral action;

(3) appropriate technology for health; and
(4) community involvement.

According to WHO's definition to which all governments have agreed, "appropriate" means that the technology is, as well as economically feasible, not only scientifically sound but also socially acceptable to those on whom it is used and to those who use it.

The International Conference on Primary Health Care held at Alma Ata in 1978 declared that the key to health for all is primary health care. It is not by chance that the first of the eight essential programme elements of primary health care is education of people concerning prevailing health problems and methods of preventing and controlling them. Nor indeed is it by chance that education of people is the first element, for if governments with all their sectors and people in all walks of life are to act in partnership for the improvement of health they must first understand how this can best be achieved. They must understand how to promote health, how to prevent and control disease, how to identify illness and treat and care for the sick and rehabilitate them as necessary.

As you know, the International Conference at Alma Ata issued a Declaration which stated that governments have responsibility for the health of their people and that they have to fulfil that responsibility by adequate health and social measures. This is in addition to another important part of the Declaration, which states that people have the right and duty to participate individually and collectively in the planning and implementation of their health care.

Thus, today, I turn to you who have both national and international responsibility for carrying out the strategy for health for all. As you know, the Health Assembly last year adopted a global strategy for the prevention and control of AIDS, a strategy that is fully consonant with the global strategy for health for all. The fight against AIDS, the global strategy for conducting that fight, follow the principles I have just mentioned regarding the strategy for health for all and primary health care.

I shall start with political commitment. I humbly submit that you, the ministers of health, using WHO's policy and strategy framework, have responsibility for ensuring the political commitment of your governments as a whole in the fight against AIDS.

You, the ministers of health, have responsibility for ensuring the coordinated action of all the sectors concerned in your country – the ministries of education, culture, the interior, finance, information, and others, all of which have important roles in the national plan to fight AIDS.

You, the ministers of health, have responsibility for ensuring that your programmes for the prevention and control of AIDS are indeed based on appropriate technology. That such technology is scientifically sound means that it includes the social and behavioural sciences; that it is socially acceptable means that it includes consideration of social, cultural, and educational factors. Public information on AIDS must be accepted by your people, by the different groups of your people as well as by health workers. And, of course, you have to take into account your own economic situation in devising feasible plans.

You, the ministers of health, are the guardians of primary health care in your countries and of the important educational component I mentioned a few moments ago. I need not impress upon you the importance of the right kind of communication with the different groups of people in your country to whom I have just referred. I believe that you will benefit from research and development studying optimal ways of communicating with different groups – the media, the public, health workers, risk groups, and the like. Your WHO stands ready to support you in such research and development.

Let us remember that the *all* in health for all means *all* and not just a few. As HIV-positive people and AIDS patients belong to the *all*, they are entitled to humane and understanding care just like any other people. WHO has just issued a brochure on the social aspects of AIDS prevention and control programmes which, I believe, will be most useful to you in providing guiding principles for such care.

To those of you who, as part of the global fight against AIDS, are in a position to support other countries, need I remind you of WHO's principle of enlightened bilateralism, that of supporting other countries in line with the global strategy to combat AIDS, which you adopted last May at the World Health Assembly and which, I hope, governs your own national AIDS programme? Of course, in supporting other countries you have to take into account their political, social, economic, and cultural circumstances.

WHO is now 40 years old. When it was 30, we spoke together of a dream, of health for all, of all for health. AIDS is not just another barrier to achieving that dream. The fight against AIDS is a fight for health. AIDS is a symbol of the profound global interdependence which is the special knowledge, the profound insight, of our time. AIDS teaches us yet again about the cultural, social, economic, and political dimensions to health. It shows us precisely how discrimination, marginalization, and stigmatization are themselves threats to public health. Easy solutions – no. Long-term commitment to the health of individuals through the combination of what they can, and must, do for themselves and what society only can do – yes.

This Summit gives us all a precious, doubly precious, opportunity. We shall be shown what others have done to inform and educate about AIDS. We shall see through their work how we can best proceed, if we have not already done so. And we shall, through the fact of our meeting together, through our commitment to the global AIDS strategy, draw strength from common purpose.

So I humbly submit that, by using your World Health Organization, its policies, and its strategies wisely, courageously, and vigorously, you will demonstrate that *a global effort can and will stop AIDS.*

PART I

AIDS – A Global Challenge

A global problem – a global response. AIDS has become a great and powerful symbol for a world threatened by its divisions, East and West, North and South. In a deep and remarkable way, the child with AIDS is the world's child; the man or woman dying of AIDS has become the world's image of our own mortality; AIDS is also uncertainty and the unknown. Yet we face responsibility for this day and these lives. Against AIDS we have set our common course – the global AIDS strategy.

JONATHAN MANN
Director, Global Programme on AIDS
World Health Organization, Geneva.

In the absence of medical defences against AIDS, public education is the main weapon in the fight to limit the spread of infection. Only by influencing personal behaviour and lifestyles can we hope to minimize the ravages of AIDS throughout our population.

JOHN MOORE
Secretary of State for Social Services,
United Kingdom of Great Britain and Northern Ireland.

Global AIDS: Epidemiology, Impact, Projections, Global Strategy

JONATHAN MANN*

Your Royal Highness, Mr President, Ministers, Colleagues, Ladies and Gentlemen,

It is amazing, and humbling, to realize that in the late 1970s the human immunodeficiency virus (HIV) was spreading silently – unrecognized and unnoticed – around the world; that by 1981, when AIDS was first recognized, cases had already occurred on several continents, and that the worldwide scope of HIV infection and AIDS was not fully realized until the mid-1980s. Yet, although HIV infection and AIDS stole a march on us, the global response has been rapid – the global AIDS strategy was designed and adopted, and in the past year we have witnessed an extraordinary and unprecedented global mobilization to prevent and control the disease.

To describe global AIDS it has been useful to divide the problem into three separate yet interdependent epidemics: of infection with HIV; of the disease AIDS; and of the reaction and response – social, cultural, economic, and political – to the HIV and AIDS epidemics. This analysis permits us to focus separately on each element and also emphasizes that the third epidemic, that of the reaction, is as much a part of the pathology of AIDS as the virus itself.

On the basis of the available information, we believe that HIV is an *old* if not ancient virus, of unknown geographical origin. The recent history – the current epidemic of HIV infection, the pandemic of global scope – appears to have started in the mid-1970s. From the mid-1970s to the present, we believe that several million people have become infected with HIV. Today, basing ourselves on the available information, we estimate that between 5 and 10 million persons in the world are infected with HIV. To be more precise in our estimation, more valid HIV prevalence data at the national level will be needed. Here we face a very difficult problem, for it has not yet been possible to determine the number of HIV-infected people in any individual

* Director, Global Programme on AIDS, World Health Organization, Geneva.

country. This task is urgent, for these national estimates are needed to provide the scientific basis for predicting the number of AIDS cases that can be expected during the next several years, for targeting preventive programmes, and for determining whether, where, and to what extent HIV infection is increasing in the population. They will also allow us to measure the effectiveness of preventive efforts.

Throughout the world HIV is transmitted in the same basic ways: through sex and blood, and from infected mother to child. Although variations exist regarding, for example, the dominant mode of sexual spread (heterosexual or homosexual) or the principal route of blood transmission (sharing of needles by intravenous drug users or re-use of contaminated needles for medical injections), the fundamental unity of HIV transmission must be emphasized. Despite intense international scientific scrutiny, no evidence has emerged to suggest any other modes of HIV transmission. Nor is there any evidence for any inherent racial or ethnic resistance to HIV infection or to the pathogenic effects of the virus.

The transformation of the first epidemic, that of HIV infection, into the second epidemic, of AIDS, is also becoming clearer. Our knowledge necessarily remains limited to the brief period, a decade or less, during which it has been possible to observe the state of health of HIV-infected persons. Studies of HIV-infected people have consistently shown that the risk of developing the disease AIDS increases with the length of time they are infected. Expressed in cumulative terms, in the first five years after infection between 10% and 30% develop AIDS; according to some studies, nearly 40% will develop AIDS after seven or eight years. In addition to AIDS itself, other HIV-related illnesses may occur, including persistent generalized lymphadenopathy, the AIDS-related complex (ARC), and neurological disease. Thus, in the first five years, AIDS-related illnesses may occur in 25–50% of infected persons in addition to those who develop AIDS. We do not know whether all those infected will ultimately develop AIDS; only the passage of time will clarify the final and complete outcome of HIV infection.

The long delay of years and perhaps decades between HIV infection and disease is of critical importance. Thus, all AIDS cases in 1988 and nearly all in 1989 will occur in people already infected today and probably several years ago.

By 12 January 1988, a total of 75 392 AIDS cases had been officially reported to WHO from 130 countries around the world. Of the reported cases, 75% are from 42 countries in the Americas, 12% from 27 European countries, 12% from 38 African countries, and the remaining 1% are from 23 countries in Asia and Oceania. Forty-eight countries have reported more than 50 AIDS cases to WHO, including 18 countries from the Americas, 14 from Europe, 13 from Africa, and three from Asia and Oceania.

The number of AIDS cases reported to WHO continues to rise rapidly. In the past four years it has increased more than 15 times. Nearly 100 more countries are reporting AIDS cases today than there were four years ago. This not only illustrates the widespread awareness of AIDS but also testifies to growing openness and international co-operation. When the rate of increase, rather than the absolute number of reported cases, is examined, it is interesting to note that, although the time when the curve starts in each continent differs, the slope of the curve is quite similar.

In the best of circumstances, as many as 90% of AIDS cases actually occurring in a country will be reported to the national health authority. However, in many areas the number of cases reported is substantially less than the actual number, owing to problems in recognizing or diagnosing AIDS or in reporting cases to national authorities. Taking these factors into account, we have estimated that, since the beginning of the AIDS pandemic a little over a decade ago, the actual number of AIDS cases that have occurred worldwide is approximately 150000.

The epidemic is worldwide, yet the current stage of the HIV epidemic is not the same everywhere. Three distinct epidemiological patterns can be described. The first pattern – pattern I – involves Western Europe, North America, some areas in South America, and Australia and New Zealand. The major affected groups are homosexual and bisexual men and intravenous drug users. Sexual transmission is predominantly homosexual: over 50% of homosexual men in some urban areas are HIV-infected. Although heterosexual transmission is occurring and increasing in those areas, it accounts for a much smaller portion of sexually acquired HIV infection than homosexual transmission. In pattern I areas transmission through blood principally involves intravenous drug users. After homosexual and bisexual men, intravenous drug users account for the next largest proportion of HIV-infected persons, although in some countries the majority of AIDS cases occur among intravenous drug users. HIV transmission from blood or blood products is not a continuing problem, as blood for transfusion is screened and blood products are further treated to prevent HIV contamination. In pattern I areas most HIV infections have occurred among men; however, perinatal transmission has been documented, primarily among intravenous drug-using women and sex partners of intravenous drug-using men and among women from pattern II areas of the world.

Pattern II areas include parts of Africa – principally central, eastern and southern – and parts of the Caribbean. There, sexual transmission is predominantly heterosexual and therefore the sex ratio for AIDS cases is approximately equal. In some urban areas up to 25% of the age group 20–40 years may be HIV-infected, although substantial variation has been observed, especially between urban and rural areas. Further, from 75% to 90% of female prostitutes in some areas may be HIV-infected. In pattern II areas, transfusion of HIV-infected blood is a public health problem. Non-sterile needles, syringes, and other skin-piercing instruments undoubtedly play a role in HIV transmission, but their contribution to the overall burden of HIV infection is smaller than that of sexual transmission. Finally, as a reflection of heterosexual spread, perinatal transmission is a substantial problem; in some areas 5–15% or more of pregnant women are HIV-infected.

Pattern III areas include Asia, most of the Pacific Region, the Middle East and Eastern Europe. In those areas HIV infection seems to have appeared more recently, in the early to middle 1980s. Most AIDS cases involve homosexual or heterosexual contact or receipt of imported blood or blood products. The prevalence of HIV infection in high-risk behaviour groups such as male or female prostitutes is very low. Although HIV infection has not yet penetrated into the general population of pattern III countries, the virus is present and evidence of within-country HIV transmission is increasing.

While the modes of HIV transmission are identical, therefore, the detailed epidemiology of HIV and AIDS differs substantially around the world. Of course, the three patterns described represent a generalization, for different epidemiological patterns may coexist within a country or even within a large city. Also, the patterns are not immutable. Over time, in the absence of effective prevention strategies, the three patterns might be expected to converge. Thus, if safe blood and blood products and safe injections and other skin-piercing practices become the rule, most HIV transmission will be sexual and perinatal. In addition, regardless of which sexual group is most affected with HIV in a given area today, sexual transmission may ultimately be the rule in all groups that engage in risk behaviour.

The epidemiology of HIV infection also shapes the impact of AIDS on health in each society. In general, AIDS affects two age groups predominantly: adults of 20–40 years and infants and very young children. The impact of AIDS on young adults may be severe in both industrialized and developing countries. Throughout the world, 75–90% of HIV infections and AIDS cases are occurring in the age group 20–40 years. As a result, by 1991 in a pattern I country the mortality rate among men aged 25–34 years will increase by two-thirds owing to AIDS. By 1991 in that same country the number of deaths from AIDS among men aged 25–34 years will be greater than the total number of deaths now occurring in the group from the current four major causes of death – traffic accidents, suicide, heart disease, and cancer.

In pattern II countries a scenario can be used to describe the impact of HIV infection on health among adults. In a city of one million inhabitants, if 10% of those aged 20–50 years are HIV-infected, assuming that most have been infected fairly recently, AIDS deaths in 1988 would raise the overall adult mortality rate by one-third. By 1991, even assuming that no additional people become infected, the expected AIDS deaths will raise the adult mortality rate by over 100%.

Infants represent another vulnerable population, owing principally to transmission from infected mothers. In areas where 5% of pregnant women are HIV-infected, the increase in the infant mortality rate due to HIV would be approximately 13 per 1000, which is greater than the total infant mortality rate from all causes in many industrialized countries. In populations with higher levels of infection among pregnant women, such as 20%, increases in infant mortality of 50 per 1000 or more may be anticipated. Thus, the projected gains in infant and child health from public health efforts, including the Child Survival Initiatives, may be tragically cancelled by AIDS. The concentrated impact of HIV and AIDS on young adults and infants will cause a decline in life expectancy in many industrialized and developing countries.

The effects of AIDS go far beyond changes in health statistics. A third epidemic relentlessly follows the first two epidemics: it is the economic, social, cultural and political reaction to HIV infection and AIDS. This worldwide epidemic has only started, yet it is an integral part of the global AIDS problem.

The social impact of AIDS is linked to the selective loss of persons at a time in their lives when, socially and economically, they are highly productive. In many cultures 20–40-year-old men and women are the economic support not only of children but also of older persons, for whom the family may be the only form of social security. Thus, AIDS is a particularly dangerous threat to family life; young orphans and the elderly will be left without support.

Fear and ignorance continue to lead to tragedies for individuals, families, and entire societies. Unfortunately, as anxiety and fear cause some to blame others, AIDS has unveiled thinly disguised prejudices about race, religion, social class, sex, and nationality. As a result, AIDS now threatens free travel between countries and open international communication and exchange.

Moreover, in the process of fighting AIDS we find ourselves re-examining many differing aspects of health and the social system. Like a diagnostic test, AIDS has helped us see the inadequacies and inequities in health systems. To confront AIDS, we must look again and perhaps differently at such social problems as the prostitution of women, children and men, and intravenous drug use; we must recognize long-standing weaknesses in health care systems regarding blood, needles, and invasive practices; and we find ourself re-examining the ways we speak to, inform, and educate one another about health. AIDS remorselessly highlights our most complex problems, challenges our assumptions, and shakes our complacency.

In seeking now to forecast the future, we are limited by our incomplete knowledge. Nevertheless, from the available data we estimate that in 1988 approximately 150000 new cases of AIDS will occur, equalling the total number of cases that have so far occurred worldwide. If we adopt the conservative estimate of five million people infected today with HIV, a cumulative total of one million AIDS cases can be expected by 1991. Thus the period 1989–91 will probably witness over five times more AIDS cases than have so far occurred.

What, then, is the potential for spread of HIV? Studies of intravenous drug users, homosexual and bisexual men, and women prostitutes have shown clearly that, if the virus is present in the community and the behaviour that transmits infection is sufficiently widespread and intense, HIV can cause explosive epidemics. In addition, HIV infection is lifelong, so the virus can survive in the human population if, during the life of an infected person, it can spread to one other person. This suggests that HIV infection will perpetuate itself relatively easily unless a cure or a vaccine is discovered, and neither is likely in the next several years. Thus HIV infection is likely to remain with us for the foreseeable future.

The full impact of HIV infection will be felt over decades. The virus does not need to spread rapidly in a population to have a very marked and gradually expanding cumulative effect. The two major factors influencing the risk of individual infection are the prevalence of HIV infection and individual behaviour. We do not have precise numbers, but it is likely that several hundred million people around the world behave in ways that make them vulnerable to infection with HIV. Thus, while it has become fashionable to be reassuring and to state that AIDS will never threaten large populations, we believe that virology, immunology, sociology and epidemiology require us to take the long view, a more sombre one. Let us remember that we are still in the early phases of a global epidemic of which the first decade gives every rational reason for concern about the global future of AIDS.

A global problem – a global response. AIDS has become a great and powerful symbol for a world threatened by its divisions, East and West, North and South. In a deep and remarkable way, the child with AIDS is the world's child; the man or woman dying of AIDS has become the world's image of our own mortality; AIDS is also uncertainty and the unknown. Yet we face responsibility for this day and these lives. Against AIDS we have set our common course – the global AIDS strategy.

The global AIDS strategy has three objectives:

- to prevent HIV infection
- to reduce the personal and social impact of HIV infection and to

care for those already infected with HIV and for those who have
AIDS
- to unify national and international efforts.

The global strategy is based on the following principles:

- public health must be protected
- human rights must be respected and discrimination against
  infected persons prevented
- we know enough now to prevent the spread of HIV, even without
  a vaccine
- education is the key to AIDS prevention, because HIV transmission can be prevented through informed and responsible
  behaviour
- AIDS control requires a sustained social and political commitment
- all countries need a comprehensive national AIDS programme,
  integrated into national health systems and linked within a global
  network
- systematic monitoring and evaluation will ensure that the global
  strategy can adapt and grow stronger with time.

The first objective, preventing HIV transmission, is achievable precisely because HIV is transmitted through the behaviour of individuals
and through a few recognized health care procedures.

Individual behaviour is responsible for most HIV transmission. It
requires the active participation of two persons; therefore the chain of
transmission can be broken by a change in the behaviour of either the
infected or the non-infected person. For that reason the proper focus
of prevention is behaviour, not infection status. To prevent HIV transmission we must inform and educate so as to obviate the adoption of
risk behaviour or to help people with such behaviour to abandon it or
modify it. For that task a four-part information and education programme is needed: for the general public, for target groups, for specific
individuals, and for health workers.

Programmes for the general public alert the public and inform them
about AIDS. For the programmes to succeed the media must be well
informed and supportive. But the behaviour involved in AIDS transmission is private, hidden from others, or frankly disapproved of by
many societies. Since we cannot know who already practises or may go
on to risk behaviour, everyone should be given information and educated about AIDS. Programmes for the general public also establish
AIDS as a legitimate national issue worthy of discussion and action.
But broad public information campaigns do not and should not be
expected to produce a rapid or sustained behaviour change. The need
to address an entire population – young and old, rich and poor, women

and men, educated and uneducated – inevitably makes a broad public programme a blunt instrument.

Not everyone is at equal risk of HIV infection so information and education, like any health intervention, should be especially targeted where it is most needed. We therefore need to discover more about the private behaviour of people. This must be done carefully, with empathy and sensitivity, otherwise vital information will be hidden and nothing useful will be learned. The information and education of target groups must involve their active participation in all phases of the programme – planning, implementing and evaluating. The alternative to working with the people it is intended to educate is dismal failure. If people believe that AIDS is a curable disease they will not use condoms. If intravenous drug users do not understand the words we use to describe needles, syringes, and other drug equipment they cannot learn about prevention. If adolescents are convinced that AIDS is being used to deprive them of sexual freedom, they may refuse to listen to prevention messages and even counter-react in ways that further endanger their lives. It is important to recognize that "we", whoever we are and regardless of our experience, do not know how best to educate "them". We need an alliance, a dialogue, not a monologue. There is evidence from around the world that, when people from target groups are asked to become involved in AIDS information and education programmes, they respond positively and sincerely and often with great energy and creativity.

Some individuals will need an even more personal relationship, not only to inform and educate them but also to support them in the difficult process of changing behaviour. Counselling, a key component of information and education programmes, must be organized and provided for individuals and small groups. Counselling is a more personal and intimate realm in which the person with high-risk behaviour, the person seeking voluntary HIV testing, the HIV-infected person, and families and friends can find information, understanding, and support.

The fourth information and education component concerns health workers. They must not only meet the challenge of informing and educating others, providing infected people with humane care, and ensuring the safety of health care procedures, but also contribute actively, through personal and community leadership, to forming an enlightened public opinion.

Such are the four components of national information and education programmes. Yet by themselves such programmes are not enough. Prevention cannot be sustained by information alone; information and education programmes can succeed only if there is a supportive social environment and if certain health and social services are made available.

A supportive social environment includes tolerance towards and avoidance of discrimination against th..se who are infected. They, and others who need help to stop risk behaviour, are also part of our society and part of us. There is no public health rationale for isolation, quarantine, or other discriminatory measures based solely on a person's HIV infection status or risk behaviour. Preventing such discrimination not only protects human rights but also helps ensure an effective AIDS programme. Discrimination and fear will undermine an entire national information and education programme. Thus discrimination itself can endanger public health.

Certain health and social services are also needed to support and strengthen people's capacity to make long-term behaviour changes. Examples of such services are: the treatment of intravenous drug users to stop drug abuse; long-term counselling for infected persons, their sexual partners, and their families; voluntary HIV-testing; and making condoms available. Good intentions are not enough. How realistic is HIV control among intravenous drug users if there are no treatment programmes for drug abuse? How likely is long-term behaviour change to be achieved without long-term access to counselling, support, and advice? How likely is condom use if condoms are too expensive, of poor quality, or simply not available?

Thus national efforts to prevent HIV transmission by means of behaviour change include a four-part information and education programme, a supportive social environment, and associated health and social services. Each is essential; the lack of any component will dramatically reduce the national capacity to prevent transmission.

The second objective of the global AIDS strategy is to reduce the personal and social effects of HIV infection. This means providing humane care, of a quality not inferior to that for other diseases, for those with HIV infection, and counselling, social support, and services for those infected but not ill. Reducing the social effects also requires a broad social and political commitment, the strength to reject simplistic solutions for AIDS control, and the will to ensure participation of the entire health and social sector in an active programme "Against AIDS – For Health".

The third objective of the global AIDS strategy is to unify national and international efforts against AIDS. The year 1987 was one of AIDS mobilization at the national and global level. There is simply no parallel to what has been accomplished in 1987. In that year many countries stood forth against AIDS. Those countries were characterized by strong public health leadership and frankness and openness about AIDS. In each such country the words "historic" and "unprecedented" were often heard, for they best described the dimension, creativity, and courage of the AIDS information and education programmes. At the centre of each such programme ministers of health and public health leaders spoke to a larger and much more interested public than other health matters in the past had received, and obtained the political support needed to make openness a reality. Before turning to the future we salute those public health leaders and their accomplishments.

In 1987 we saw evidence that all – heterosexual men and women, homosexual and bisexual men, prostitutes, intravenous drug users, adolescents – can learn and that all are capable of changing their behaviour to protect themselves from AIDS. In 1987 we saw that information and education have the potential to succeed against AIDS as no health education programme has succeeded before. Yet, despite some early successes in informing large populations about AIDS, in changing high-risk behaviours in certain groups, in establishing counselling programmes, and in training and educating health workers, it is too early for any sense of relief, too soon for self-satisfaction. Quite the contrary!

In 1988 the challenge will be fourfold. We must:

- open fully the channels of communication in each society, so as to inform and educate people more broadly and intensively
- through information, education, and social leadership, create a spirit of social tolerance, so as to combat the discrimination that threatens public health
- establish a social and political commitment, to ensure that the health and social services needed will be available to sustain changes in behaviour; the precious fruit of education must not be allowed to rot from neglect or lack of support
- ensure, where it has not yet been done, the safety of blood and blood products, injections, and other skin-piercing procedures performed within or outside the health system.

In a few short years our technical understanding of AIDS has progressed rapidly. We know a great deal about a virus we did not even suspect existed ten years ago. Yet, perhaps more importantly, the global, social, and personal significance of AIDS is coming rapidly to the forefront, and human understanding of this situation is the basis of our common fight. We have a global strategy against a global disease and we see that, to an extraordinary degree, the fight against AIDS is a fight for health. AIDS must be combated on its own terms, by achieving changes in behaviour and by ensuring safe practices in the health system. Yet, through this particular disease, we are led inevitably and irresistibly to larger and more general problems and issues. We are committed not just against AIDS, but for health; not just for today, but for decades to come. AIDS is a threat, but through it we may realize the promise of health promotion and the potential of primary health care, so that we may thereby come yet closer to the dream of health for all.

Our opportunity, brought so clearly into focus by this Summit, is truly historic. We live in a world threatened by unlimited destructive force, yet we share a vision of creative potentiality: personal, national, and international. The dream of health for all is not new, but the circumstances and the opportunity are of our time alone. The global AIDS problem speaks eloquently of the need for communication, for the sharing of information and experience, and for mutual support. AIDS shows us once again that silence, exclusion, and isolation, whether of individuals, groups, or nations, create a danger for all of us.

Against AIDS, shall we dominate the disease, all three epidemics, through information-sharing and international cooperation, or shall we allow the disease and the fears it unleashes to dominate us? Against AIDS, shall we prevail together, or shall we split and cast into the shadows those persons, groups, and nations that are affected?

During this global summit on AIDS we shall hear about examples of excellent work that has been done, of an already evident impact, and of the creativity called forth by this new challenge. The tools for prevention are available to all and await their full, combined, and vigorous use in all countries. We know how next to proceed. The global AIDS strategy, fully applied in every country, will start the sequence that leads, through behaviour change, to slowing down the spread of the AIDS virus itself. Thus, in this year of 1988 it is possible to enter a new era in our confrontation with AIDS. The vision of this world Summit unites us all. With confidence in our collective course, let us proceed from this Summit to make history together.

Modes of Transmission: the Basis for Prevention Strategies

SIR DONALD ACHESON*

Your Royal Highness, Mr President, Ministers, Colleagues, Ladies and Gentlemen,

I regard it as a great responsibility and privilege to have been given the opportunity to address such a distinguished audience, gathered from the four corners of the earth, on this topic.

I should like to take as my starting-point the quotation which you see at the beginning of your programme. It is taken from an address by my Secretary of State to the United Nations General Assembly in October 1987, where he said "In the absence of medical defences against AIDS, public education is the main weapon in the fight to limit the spread of infection. Only by influencing personal behaviour and lifestyles can we hope to minimize the ravages of AIDS throughout our population."

Thus the nature of the problem which this summit conference is addressing is such that it is necessary to talk, in simple practical terms understandable to all, about aspects of human behaviour so intimate that five years ago they were barely spoken about in many parts of the world except in whispers. I shall also be referring to aspects of human behaviour which are not universally acceptable and which in many places are beyond the law. As a public health doctor whose duty is to help all people preserve and improve their health I make no judgements, but I hope you will recognize that I am sensitive to the moral and social issues which lie at the root of this epidemic. I crave your indulgence and, if I give offence to anyone, forgiveness.

Your Royal Highness, we are dealing with a virus which we must regard as potentially lethal to all who are infected with it. While treatment can reduce suffering and provide support, no cure is in sight. Nor is a vaccine available which would render people injected with it immune from infection. For the time being our only weapon is to devise

* Chief Medical Officer, Department of Health and Social Security, United Kingdom of Great Britain and Northern Ireland.

14

and implement strategies which will stop the passage of the virus from one person to another and thus stop the spread of the epidemic.

To do this we must base our strategy on a knowledge of how the virus is and is not transmitted. In fact, the routes of transmission can be described quite briefly. They are threefold. The virus is transmitted by:

- penetrative sexual intercourse with an infected person
- inoculation of infected blood
- spread from an infected mother to the unborn fetus, to the baby as it is delivered, or during breast-feeding.

It is equally important to know how the virus is *not* transmitted. It is *not* transmitted by social contact, for example within families, nor by food or water, nor by insect bites, nor by contact with telephones, toilet seats, or used clothes, nor by contact at work, except in a few rare instances in health care workers.

The object of our preventive policy is to slow down and if possible stop transmission of the virus.

Sexual intercourse

The most important way in which the virus is passed on is during penetrative sexual intercourse with an infected person. Transmission can undoubtedly occur as a result of peno-vaginal intercourse from male to female and female to male. The more partners, the greater the risk. It seems likely that other inflammatory genital disease and in particular genital ulcer, which is frequent in some parts of the world, increases the risk of transmission.

Transmission also undoubtedly occurs as a result of peno-anal intercourse between men and between men and women. Again, as one might expect, the greater the number of partners the greater the risk. There is substantial and consistent evidence that amongst homosexual men the partner who receives the sperm is much more at risk than the other.

The risk of infection by sexual intercourse can clearly be avoided by life-long celibacy or by restricting intercourse to a mutually monogamous relationship with an uninfected person. In practical terms, however, it is obvious that by itself such advice is insufficient to meet the needs of everyone. The risk can be reduced by reducing the number of partners and by the use of a condom of high quality throughout intercourse. It also seems likely that steps taken to eliminate genital ulcer and perhaps other inflammatory genital diseases would reduce the rate of spread of the virus.

Prostitutes of both sexes are vulnerable to infection with HIV and can themselves pass on the virus. It is crucial for their own sakes and those of their clients that they insist on the use of condoms.

With regard to types of sexual activity other than penetrative inter-course, there is at present no sound evidence which implicates them in the transmission of this virus. There is no convincing evidence that genito-oral sex or kissing transmits the infection.

Blood to blood

HIV may also be transmitted when infected blood or blood products are introduced into the blood of another person. Just as people who have become infected sexually may transmit the infection to others through blood, so people infected through blood may transmit the virus to their sexual partners, and infected women to their unborn children.

In the United Kingdom and a number of other developed countries, by far the most important means of transmission by blood is through the infected syringe needle and other paraphernalia of people who inject illegal narcotic and other drugs. While the intravenous route is the usual one, subcutaneous injections are also sometimes used by drug abusers and should also be avoided. Research has shown that the risk of infection is related to the frequency with which the person injects and with which he or she shares equipment with others.

Put in their simplest terms, the principles underlying risk avoidance and reduction in this field can be summarized in the following sentences:

If you do not abuse drugs, do not begin.
If you abuse drugs, do not inject.
If you inject, use sterile equipment and never share.

I do not have to underline the difficulties in reducing the rate of spread by these means. It is necessary to develop a set of policies which, in addition to the correction of social conditions conducive to drug abuse and reduction of the supply of and demand for such drugs, will encourage those who are already abusing drugs to come forward and to change their behaviour in a direction which is safer for others and safer for themselves. This will involve a number of controversial decisions relating to groups of people who are in many parts of the world outside the law and alienated, and who often finance their habit by prostitution. The key is to encourage these people to come forward for education and treatment. But for those who cannot or will not stop injecting, consideration will also have to be given to the propriety of providing sterile equipment to render them less of a risk to others. Those who are infected should be advised on how to reduce the risk of infecting their sexual partners by abstinence or the correct use of condoms.

Because drug abuse is illegal, prisons often have a relatively high prevalence of HIV infection. The problems of possible spread of the virus within prisons and after the prisoner is released must be faced.

Unsterile syringes, needles, and other medical equipment may also transmit HIV when used for the administration of antibodies, vaccines, and other legitimate medicaments by doctors and nurses as well as traditional practitioners. Frequent medical injections have been shown to be a risk factor for HIV in African children and, judging by experience with the transmission of other virus infections (e.g., hepatitis B and Ebola fever), are likely also to be a factor in adults. The abolition of this risk requires not only the supply of appropriate sterile equipment but also programmes of training for health care workers and for traditional healers. It is a catastrophe if a patient is given an injection which cures gonorrhoea but transmits HIV. Although no known cases have yet been reported of transmission of the virus by these means, other procedures which involve penetration of the skin, including tattooing, acupuncture, and penetration of the skin for cosmetic treatment, are a potential means of transmission and should always be carried out with sterile equipment. This requires the development of appropriate policies and the provision of guidance to those who use these procedures.

It is a tragic fact that blood transfusion still remains an important means of transmission of HIV in some parts of the world. The risk of infection can be markedly reduced by testing all blood donors for HIV antibodies. In those countries where the prevalence of HIV infection is largely limited to specific subgroups of the population, it is important also to invite these people not to present themselves as donors. Similar precautions are necessary in respect of donations of tissue for transplantation and of sperm for artificial insemination.

There are few countries in the world where unnecessary transfusion of blood does not occur. HIV infection is an additional good reason for health authorities and the medical profession in all countries to stop unnecessary transfusions of blood. In countries where HIV infection is prevalent it would be prudent to consider limiting blood transfusions to situations where it is life-saving. As far as the use of factors VIII and IX in the treatment of haemophilia is concerned, screening of donors, together with proper heat treatment, has eliminated the risk of HIV infection.

Eleven cases in the world are known where the virus has been transmitted from infected patients to people nursing them. They have involved either injury with an infected needle or gross contamination of the skin or mucous membranes of the nurse. In most cases the skin of the health care worker who became infected was damaged in some way. In one case there was gross contamination of the nurse, who was untrained and did not wear gloves. While these cases are a reason for anxiety and remind us of the need for health care workers to follow the highest practicable standards of hygiene in dealing with all patients, it is reassuring that a follow-up of many hundreds of health care workers who have suffered an injury as a result of an infected needle has shown that less than 1% have subsequently been found to be infected. Sound hygienic medical and nursing practice and extreme care in handling sharp instruments and disposing of them are the keys to risk reduction in this area.

Perinatal transmission

Tragically, about half of the babies born to mothers infected with HIV turn out themselves to be infected. The evidence so far is that they do badly. Much has still to be learned about the means by which the virus enters the blood of these babies. However, it is clear that they may be infected before or during delivery. The breast milk of infected women has been found to contain the virus. Three instances have been reported where mothers who became infected as a result of a blood transfusion given to them during the delivery of the baby subsequently infected the baby during breast-feeding.

What can be done to reduce the frequency of these tragic births? Best of all is to prevent women of reproductive age becoming infected. In countries where the virus is largely limited to particular subgroups, policies to reduce the rate of infection of women of reproductive age must be prepared and implemented. Where the male partner is known to be already infected, abstinence or the use of condoms where these are acceptable is the only means at our disposal. Women presenting in early pregnancy may be offered testing for HIV antibodies. In cultures where abortion is acceptable this gives them the opportunity to consider this option, although it must be recognized that, on average, an infected mother has an even chance of giving birth to an infection-free baby.

Where a safe alternative type of feeding is easily available it may be prudent to recommend that infected mothers should not breast-feed, but not where a safe alternative is not available.

Conclusion

In conclusion, I wish to make three points. The first is that it must be obvious from what I have said that, if we are to succeed in slowing down or stopping the spread of this fearful virus, rapid, profound, and widespread changes in human behaviour will have to take place. The dissemination of correct information is the key to changes in attitudes; and changes in attitudes are the key to changes in behaviour and the learning of new skills. Correct information, and its delivery in unambiguous, simple, and comprehensible terms suitably expressed for the needs of a wide variety of groups – older children and adolescents, adult men and women, prostitutes, drug abusers, and so on – is the foundation of all that follows.

To bring about such changes is, as must be abundantly clear, far beyond the capacity or skill of the medical profession alone, or of scientists or their allies in the field of health care. One only has to remember that, even where there is an effective and simple treatment available for a sexually transmitted disease like syphilis or gonorrhoea, we have not succeeded in controlling the disease. Sexually transmitted diseases have their origins in the cultures of the societies in which we live. Medical scientists will accomplish nothing without the help and guidance of society as a whole, not just politicians and religious leaders.

My second point relates to the difficulties associated with practical advice regarding risk reduction. It is right to advise people to stick to one faithful partner, but is it right to advise that if they do not they should use a condom? It is right to advise people not to abuse drugs by injection, but is it right to encourage and support those who cannot stop so that they become less of a hazard to others? Each politician and each private citizen here today will have his views on these points. But it is the duty of the public health doctor to put before all of you the grave nature of this infection and to warn you that we cannot guarantee that an easy scientific solution to it will soon, or indeed ever, be developed. It is in this context that the issues I have just mentioned should be decided.

My final point is one of hope. All of us can take encouragement from the fact that those groups who so far have been at highest risk and whom we have been able to study have changed their behaviour in the direction of safety, and that the rate of spread of infection has declined within them.

PART II

AIDS Prevention Through Health Promotion

National AIDS information programmes for the general public

This section of the proceedings describes how four countries – Brazil, France, Uganda, and the United Kingdom of Great Britain and Northern Ireland – have organized national AIDS health promotion activities, using multiple media and communication techniques to inform and educate the general public about HIV infection and AIDS.

Dr Anthony Meyer, Chief, Health Promotion, WHO Global Programme on AIDS, introduces the section with an outline of the place and scope of health promotion in the control and prevention of HIV infection and AIDS.

Introduction

A photograph of a child with AIDS appeared on the cover of a major news magazine. Her father became infected with HIV while injecting drugs into himself with a contaminated needle and syringe. Her mother was then infected through sexual transmission. The child was born infected with AIDS from her mother. Drug use, sex, and perinatal transmission forged a silent but deadly chain which now threatens her life.

We can break that chain, not through a cure or a vaccine – either of which may be years away – but through information and education. Information and education on AIDS are fundamental to prevention, for the simple reason that AIDS is transmitted by specific acts that are largely subject to individual control. Personal action is the fundamental measure in stopping AIDS.

However, information also has a potential for harm. Too often the first news of AIDS is sensationalized, stigmatizing, horrifying, or distorted. First impressions are powerful and, if uncorrected, may persist and deepen into misleading beliefs and myths about AIDS. Such beliefs and myths may harm people and threaten public health by leading to denial, blame, helplessness, and passivity:

- *denial* that AIDS is a global problem with the potential to affect not only the life of homosexual men, prostitutes, or intravenous drug users, but also the life of everyone
- *blame*, in which AIDS is someone else's fault and therefore someone else's problem
- *helplessness*, arising from the belief that people cannot protect themselves and that others determine whether a person will be infected
- *passivity*, in the belief that, until a vaccine or cure is found, nothing can be done to prevent AIDS, that people are powerless to protect themselves.

---

* Chief, Health Promotion, Global Programme on AIDS, World Health Organization, Geneva.

This progression of denial, blame, helplessness, and passivity leaves people confused and vulnerable to AIDS infection.

The WHO Global Programme on AIDS is based on the belief that through accurate information and intensive education the spread of AIDS can be stopped. This belief is grounded in the view that:

- people learn when they are motivated to do so
- when people learn they can use what they have learned and integrate it into their own lives
- individuals are influenced in their behaviour by others.

Thus, people who *have learned*, who *wish to use* what they have learned, who are *influenced positively* by others, and who *have the opportunity* and support to *modify their behaviour* will do so. Examples of such learning and change in behaviour are to be found all around us and are reflected in our personal habits, our choice of food and drink, our beliefs about our bodies and how to protect our health.

The challenge to our world, a world living in the shadow of AIDS, is clear and urgent. To prevent the spread of AIDS, we must seek to influence positively the behaviour of individuals and groups, using our most effective strategies, what we know about AIDS, and what we can learn about information and education, society and culture. National AIDS prevention and control programmes throughout the world will succeed or fail to the extent that they meet this challenge. Presented with the unprecedented opportunity to prevent AIDS from becoming the massive pandemic it clearly has the potential to become, we must look to the future, when we will have to ask ourselves these questions:

- *Did* we inform?
- *Did* we educate?
- *Did* we have the courage to do enough?

Experience throughout the world in relation to such public health challenges as the prevention of heart disease, the reduction of tobacco use, the control of diarrhoeal disease, the promotion of immunization, and family planning provides us with information and education techniques that can be used against AIDS. Although they have many names and academic descriptions, we prefer to call them "health promotion". Health promotion provides a rational and systematic way to plan, implement, and monitor and evaluate information and education programmes to combat AIDS.

A solid understanding of health promotion is essential for those who direct and coordinate AIDS prevention and control programmes. Without informed support AIDS health promotion cannot succeed. Two panels during this summit meeting will focus on health promotion. The first will discuss programmes for the general public. The second will be concerned with programmes for people at risk from specific practices such as intravenous drug use and prostitution.

AIDS health promotion begins with planning. Effective planning relies on information at the local and national level. We need to know about AIDS and HIV infection, their extent and distribution – in other words, their epidemiology within the country. We need also to know about risk behaviour and those who practise risk behaviour. While the modes of HIV transmission are the same worldwide, through sex, blood, and mother-to-child transmission, we need to learn about the frequency and distribution of such risk behaviour as the use of contaminated needles or prostitution, as well as the cultural context of such behaviour. This becomes a focus for information, services, and programmes. We must also assess people's knowledge and thinking about AIDS, its spread, and its prevention. We must determine which channels for information and education are most appropriate:

- the *media* – newspapers and journals, radio, television
- institutional channels – voluntary societies, religious organizations,
- schools, government agencies
- interpersonal channels – teachers, health workers, counsellors, social workers.

Finally, we must decide on the content of the information, the vital organizations and systems, and the cost.

Brief information campaigns and uncoordinated efforts would not be sufficient and would waste resources. A plan for AIDS health promotion covering several years is needed:

- to maintain a clear and consistent focus on specific audiences
- to reinforce the information through a variety of channels and messages often repeated.

The health promotion plan should:

- be an integral part of the national AIDS plan
- involve target audiences in the design and testing of programmes intended for them
- include a monitoring and evaluation process.

Implementing AIDS health promotion requires commitment and sustained support. It is inevitable, given the subject, that controversies will arise over materials, messages, and strategies. We have already seen that, in countries using aggressive images to alert the public about AIDS, programmes are criticized for being too shocking. In countries with more subtle strategies programmes are criticized for being too cautious and timid. There is no single correct approach for all the countries of the world, and within a country the right approach for one group may be totally unsuitable for another. The challenge is to be explicit and clear, to involve those to be educated, and to be attuned to the concerns, strengths, and limitations of those you are trying to reach, so that the intended audience will learn to protect itself from HIV infection.

If we had known enough a few years ago, the story of the child with AIDS might be different today. Health promotion might have provided her father or mother with the information and education they needed to protect themselves and her against AIDS. How much effort would have been enough? Only an effort on that level will be enough to stop AIDS.

Evaluation of AIDS health promotion is an important part of the overall plan. It is not an academic exercise, but a way of improving the programme. Which strategies work best to reduce high-risk behaviour? Which institutional networks should be strengthened? Success in health promotion must be measured, lessons must be learned. Fear of evaluation must be overcome, for without dispassionate evaluation we may not recognize effective strategies and we risk perpetuating ineffective programmes. It is the special task of AIDS programmes everywhere to continue to learn even as we act. We are all pressed for time and resources, but even a modest and brief evaluation effort is better than no evaluation at all.

To help meet the personal and social challenge of health promotion, the WHO Global Programme on AIDS is providing support to countries around the world. This support consists of the following major elements:

(1) Technical expertise in planning, implementing, monitoring, and evaluating health promotion. Technical and financial support to national AIDS programmes can help in the planning of health promotion, the creation and testing of materials, and the development of practical ways of monitoring and evaluating.

(2) A series of publications under the general title "AIDS Prevention through Health Promotion". The volume entitled "Folio" contains representative health promotional materials from all over the world. A technical guide for AIDS health promotion, intended for national and district-level health communicators and national AIDS committees, will be available shortly.

(3) An exchange programme to share information and experience from around the world. The Global Programme on AIDS is supporting regional and global AIDS health promotion materials exchange centres, publishing the AIDS Health Promotion Exchange newsletter, and organizing meetings and consultations on health promotion.

(4) Practical monitoring and evaluation strategies in AIDS health promotion.

Many, indeed most, countries are already engaged in AIDS prevention through health promotion. This reflects the strength and scope of the global mobilization against AIDS. It has taken courageous leadership to initiate such programmes, often in the face of public scepticism, denial, and antagonism. Even more courage will now be required to develop AIDS health promotion plans and ensure their implementation and critical evaluation. Political support and commitment will be fundamental to the success of AIDS health promotion. With the will and determination to act we can overcome ignorance, denial, and helplessness in relation to AIDS and provide the confident leadership needed.

National AIDS Information Programme in France

ALAIN POMPIDOU

Professor Alain Pompidou is adviser on AIDS to Mrs Michèle Barzach, Minister of Health and the Family, France, and coordinator of the French National AIDS Programme. His paper outlines the information and education measures taken by the Government of France (1) to promote, especially among the young, a sense of social and individual responsibility for preventing transmission of HIV infection, and (2) to train health care and social services staff in AIDS control measures.

By the end of 1987 the number of cases of AIDS recorded in France had reached 3 073, or 56 per million inhabitants. France is therefore the European country most severely affected by this new viral infection. This was one of the reasons that impelled Mrs Barzach, Minister of Health and the Family, to set up a coordination structure as early as January 1987. The Minister also created an advisory committee to advise her on the important decisions to be taken in the fight against AIDS. Its members include scientists, specialists in ethics, education, communication, and leisure, and representatives of firms, insurance companies, and the clergy.

The national coordinator is responsible for:

- ensuring that the activities of the different ministries are complementary
- coordinating international research and cooperation
- establishing ties with private associations and organizations, including nongovernmental organizations, foundations, and industrial groups.

This made it possible to carry out a large-scale information programme while at the same time organizing preventive measures:

- by setting up widely accessible screening facilities
- by encouraging the use of condoms and controlling the quality of the brands available
- by making syringes available for sale without either a prescription or control of identity

- by care facilities
- by research
- by international cooperation.

The AIDS information campaign is therefore part of a balanced and global policy which takes into account the different aspects involved.

The national information programme was carried out in three stages:

- informing health professionals
- making both the general public and young people more aware of the problem
- training the personnel of the information outlets used.

The first two stages used a health education structure, the Health Education Committee, already in existence and responsible to the Ministry.

Informing health professionals

It is part of the doctor's role to reassure the anxious and to make the indifferent more aware of health risks. It therefore seemed vital as a first step to direct our information campaign at doctors. The campaign was carried out with the help of a million copies of documents published by the Health Education Committee and booklets edited by the group in charge of further education for medical personnel (UNAFORMEC).

The regularly updated data published in the *Weekly epidemiological bulletin* were backed up by special editions in the medical press and, in the field, by the organization of conference cycles both for hospital doctors and for doctors working in large towns.

Informing the general public, and young people in particular

The AIDS campaign was made a recognized national movement in 1987 and its aims were precisely defined:

- to provide people with scientific information that is both precise and clear
- to encourage a sense of personal responsibility rather than fear
- to provide effective means of prevention
- to ensure the coherence of the information given.

The following slogan was chosen:

"I'm not going to spread AIDS"

All the available media aids were used: radio, television, billboards, and distribution of printed material. We sent 24 million leaflets with their telephone bills to all households, and distributed 13 million brochures aimed at the general public through the social services, pharmacists, and general practitioners, and to the armed forces, universities, and the Red Cross.

A data bank was also made available through the telematic network Minitel, functioning for 24 hours a day and completely anonymous. More than 80 000 calls were recorded through this telematic network.

Finally, a specific campaign was launched with, as a target, young people of between 15 and 18 years of age. It consisted of conference debates and the preparation of audiovisual material to be distributed to all secondary schools through the rectorates.

After these two awareness campaigns, which used audiovisual communication methods for the most part, information structures are being progressively set up. They essentially concern three sectors:

- *hospitals,* especially the 22 hospitals designated as HIV information and care centres in Paris, metropolitan France, French Guyana
- *anonymous free screening centres,* which have now been set up in every department in metropolitan France and overseas
- *the associations,* especially the association AIDES, which now has outlets in most large towns.

The information being transmitted is aimed not only at doctors and the general public but also at auxiliary medical personnel and social workers.

Training the personnel of information outlets

After making the population as a whole more aware of the problem, it seemed vital to us to turn our attention to more specific targeted information based on face-to-face discussion. We then had to train the personnel of information outlets. More than 20 training programmes are now in operation, with almost 2 000 trainees, consisting of:

- auxiliary medical workers outside hospitals
- social workers
- people working in the health field
- people working with drug addicts.

The teaching is done in seminars lasting 1–3 days, providing both theoretical information and discussion of practical cases. The programmes include:

- the clinical and biological background to the infection
- screening methods
- preventive methods

- socioeconomic implications
- legal elements.

Evaluation of the information campaign

The most recent epidemiological studies show that the spread of the disease through sexual contact is on the decrease as compared with that among drug addicts. This encourages us to continue our information and prevention efforts and to concentrate even more on the fight against drug addiction, which the French Government is particularly determined to stamp out.

In one year:

- the use of voluntary or freely agreed to screening has tripled
- the use of condoms has risen by 38% and a condom quality control programme has been set up on a national scale
- the sale of syringes has more than doubled in the most exposed areas of large towns.

This finding is encouraging. We must, however, persevere in our efforts because AIDS is essentially an avoidable disease and each individual must realize that his fate is in his own hands.

Principles of health education

Before finishing, I would remind you of the principles that govern any properly thought-out health education policy:

- being informed does not necessarily mean knowing
- being aware does not necessarily mean taking steps
- deciding does not necessarily mean doing.

Informing so that there is understanding, understanding so that there is knowledge, knowing so that decisions are taken, deciding to act: it appears necessary to develop the individual's sense of responsibility during each of those stages in our health education policy. It is such a sense of responsibility, rather than obligation or duress, that leads to the most effective and widely accepted changes in behaviour among groups at risk.

The policy adopted by the French Government tries to reconcile public health protection with the observance of a certain number of fundamental principles, especially that of according to all human beings, both sick and well, the respect that is their due.

I hope that this reminder will encourage all governments concerned to join in the fight against AIDS and to persevere in their information and prevention efforts, while keeping in mind the sociocultural characteristics of the people in their charge.

Planning AIDS Education for the Public in Uganda

SAMUEL I. OKWARE

Dr Samuel I. Okware is Chairman of the National Committee for the Prevention of AIDS in Uganda and former Director of Disease Prevention and Control at the Ministry of Health. He describes how the National Committee is organized and functions and how it went about the task of planning and implementing its health promotion campaign to prevent transmission of HIV.

We are approaching the twenty-first century with uncertainties – uncertainties in our traditional values, our basic instinct for survival and our lifestyles – and all because of one of man's smallest enemies, the AIDS virus. Without a vaccine and without drugs, health promotion and education of the public are the key to interrupting the transmission of the virus. Our Ugandan programme therefore is built on that principle. The many facets of AIDS demand that health promotion and education be well planned.

Components of educational planning

What does planning of health promotion and education involve? Planning involves the setting of objectives and the selection of methods for achieving them. We must obtain resources and materials, and use them skilfully. We must check progress and modify our programmes as necessary. And we must evaluate our programmes.

The educational objectives cannot be achieved without complete openness. Nothing must be hidden. The people must be told the facts. The reason for this is that they need to be fully involved in the struggle. We were convinced that AIDS would ultimately be stopped if the people were fully educated about its nature.

Our first cases of AIDS appeared four years ago. Since that time we have learned and re-learned many lessons of planning.

Organization

How then did we plan and structure our programme? There must be only one national plan; there is no place for separate parallel programmes. To begin with, we set up a broad-based national AIDS committee with 20 members, as an appropriate forum for bringing to light the attitudes and views of different groups. It has five subcommittees, including one on health promotion and education. The national committee consists of senior professionals from the ministries of health, information, defence, and prisons, from other social service departments, and from the national university. Nongovernmental organizations, church organizations, prominent personalities in civic and private life, and traditional healers are also represented. The committee assists in policy formulation and is concerned with the complex medical, psychological, philosophical and, indeed, spiritual issues raised by AIDS.

The decisions taken by the committee are coordinated and implemented through a national AIDS control programme within the Ministry of Health. This programme has three levels. The central level provides leadership and coordination with other components and it designs, produces and supplies educational material. Implementation of the programme takes place at the district and community level. The programme is fully integrated into the existing health and social infrastructure and into primary health care.

We designed a six-month emergency plan, a two-year medium-term plan, and a five-year plan.

Definition of the problem

Planning requires the setting of clearly defined goals and objectives. The extent of the problem had to be sharply defined. The general modes of HIV transmission were well known, i.e., sex, blood, and from mother to child. But we had to determine the details of those risk factors as they applied to local circumstances. We had to determine which were the high-risk and which the low-risk groups.

We also discovered factors that seemed to be influencing the spread of the disease. We found that over 80% of cases occurred between the ages of 19 and 40 years, the peak age group for sexual activity, and 5–10% under the age of 5 years. There were virtually no cases or evidence of infection between 5 and 14 years or among the elderly (over 55 years).

Both sexes were equally affected. It also became clear that AIDS in Uganda is a disease of urban areas, where only 10% of the population live. It is rare in rural areas, with their strict traditional codes of morality. However, we know that the infection can be brought from the city to the village by city dwellers with relatives and friends in the villages.

Methods and approaches

To design suitable messages for the public we must first assess the risk behaviour of the different groups to be informed and educated. We need to discover what they believe about AIDS: from whom they get information, what their attitudes are towards risk behaviour, towards persons with AIDS and their families, and towards people who practise risk behaviour, and what among their usual practices may put them and their sexual partners at risk. For instance, one of our surveys showed that 60% of the population had first heard about AIDS from friends. This assessment of risk behaviour enables us to design interventions and messages to counter and correct misconceptions about AIDS. It also provides the baseline data against which to monitor changes resulting from health education.

Messages need to be simple and to the point, and they need to be pre-tested. They may need to be modified or replaced in the face of public criticism. We cannot afford to antagonize the people and lose their confidence.

In Uganda the message to the public is: "LOVE CAREFULLY".

The number of posters and leaflets distributed has gone up from under 2000 in the first year of the programme to over two million last year. We use all the mass media. City people have radio and television; television commercials are one of our weapons against ignorance. Most of our rural people do not have radio or television and a large proportion are illiterate. Therefore we had to use approaches that do not depend on the mass media or on literacy. We have mainly used the resistance committees, which form the backbone of the political infrastructure in the villages, to transmit simple but effective health information and education from door to door. We also use public meetings and political rallies to educate the people.

We ascertained early on that 92% of the population went to church regularly. The church is respected and accepted as an authority on moral issues. We therefore organized seminars on AIDS for the clergy, and they have been using their pulpits very extensively and very effectively to transmit the AIDS-control message. Their message to their flock is: "LOVE FAITHFULLY".

We called meetings of schoolteachers to prepare them for explaining the nature of AIDS transmission and prevention to high-school children. The children pass the message from child to child and through whispers to their parents and older relatives.

Resources

Planning must provide for the best use of our resources. Our greatest resources are human resources, the people, and their abundant good-will. The health promotion component of the national plan takes account of the potential of different groups, nongovernmental organizations, action groups, benevolent individuals – any group or individual with a contribution to make. The plan provides for integrating and coordinating their efforts and contributions with those of the national plan. It is an expression of community participation in primary health care as applied to AIDS control.

The primary focus of our health promotion and education strategy is the community, where people live and reproduce, work and play. AIDS is not just a doctor's business, or a nurse's business, or an expert's business. Everybody, everywhere, is needed to assist in every way to spread the word about AIDS.

Money, as usual, was scarce. However, it was decided to set aside separate funds for AIDS control, hence the funding of our other health programmes was not affected. We had to acknowledge our financial limitations, however. Here we called on WHO, as the global coordinating agency. With its help the Government convened a meeting of interested participating parties and funds for both the emergency and the mid-term plan were pledged. For this we are most grateful.

Monitoring and indicators of progress

Planning must be sufficiently flexible to respond to changing circumstances and interim outcomes. For this, monitoring is essential. The programme may need to be adjusted, expanded, or redirected. Indicators must be built in to help in monitoring progress.

It takes years, of course, to reduce the incidence of AIDS cases, even though transmission of the virus may be considerably reduced or even stopped. A continuing high incidence may give rise to frustration and disappointment among the public. They see that, despite everything we are doing, the number of new cases does not fall and may even rise. They may not appreciate that some of this is due to better surveillance and case detection. Today's new cases were, after all, infected many years back, some even before any programme was started.

In the long run, however, our efforts will bear fruit. Of this we are confident. And we must transmit and sustain this confidence, realistically, to the public.

Attendance at clinics for sexually transmitted diseases has already dropped considerably, from long lines in 1986 to only a few people a day in 1987. This drop in demand for the treatment of venereal diseases indicates a substantial decrease in the numbers of people who put themselves at risk of HIV infection. Private medical practitioners who thrived on treating patients with venereal diseases were the first to complain about lack of patients. Night clubs are complaining about lack of clients.

With increased public awareness, we should anticipate and prevent prejudice, disinformation, and victimization of those with AIDS. We should not wait for this to happen. Often people are wrongly informed. The press, for instance, may give distorted information. People interpret things in different ways. Such disinformation can be disastrous. Prejudice, victimization, and discrimination feed on disinformation. Both the infected and the uninfected have to be protected against disinformation and prejudice.

Health education needs to be supported by counselling for people with AIDS and their families and other close associates, as well as for those with AIDS phobia, obsessed with the fear of catching AIDS.

Programme evaluation

Finally, planning provides for the evaluation of our programme. Are our objectives and methods the right ones? Do they need to be changed? Do we need new objectives or new methods?

Are we using our resources to the best effect? Are we wasting resources? Are we making the right impact? To what extent are communities, our target groups, exercising responsibility for their own health protection and promotion?

Conclusion

The battle against AIDS must be planned and fought on many fronts. We must fight against ignorance, against prejudice, against systematic disinformation. Information and health education are the main weapons with which to fight AIDS. In a world with AIDS, life must go on. This is the real challenge to planning.

Brazil's Educational Programme on AIDS Prevention

LAIR GUERRA DE MACEDO RODRIGUES

Dr Lair Guerra de Macedo Rodrigues is Director, National Division of Sexually Transmitted Diseases and AIDS, Ministry of Health, Brazil. Of particular interest in her account of Brazil's programme is the strong intersectoral element, private and public, and the painstaking approach towards developing an active role for the Roman Catholic church in the programme.

The AIDS prevention education unit in Brazil, which is part of the National Division of Sexually Transmitted Diseases and AIDS of the Ministry of Health, works closely with other ministries in the fight against AIDS.

The Brazilian AIDS programme is directed at four broad audiences:

- health professionals
- the public at large
- groups engaging in high-risk behaviour
- adolescents.

These audiences were selected between 1985 and 1986 when results of newspaper surveys showed that they were the most affected by unfounded fears.

Health professionals

The most serious problem, one we frequently encounter in these groups, is the attitude of health professionals shown towards persons infected with HIV. They often refuse to assist patients and their families out of fear of becoming infected.

The first action the Ministry of Health took to remedy the situation was to convoke a meeting of AIDS experts in order to establish guidelines for training health professionals working in STD/AIDS clinics. The training programme began in March 1986, under the direction of a multidisciplinary team from each of the 26 states, which had been specially trained over 15 days in interpersonal skills in settings simulating the relationship between health professional and patient.

The methodology used is the training-the-trainer approach, with its multiplier effect. This type of training solved the problem partially. We are now developing new strategies to convince surgeons and haemodialysis workers that they should treat AIDS patients.

The public at large

Like the first group, the public at large suffered from misinformation conveyed by the media and reluctance to talk openly of their sexuality and their sexual practices.

In January 1986 we conducted two surveys to obtain data that would help us in developing an educational programme. For the first we employed a private advertising agency to find out which of the mass media were most commonly used by the general public. The second survey, conducted by the Folha de São Paulo newspaper in eight Brazilian cities, sought to gather information on the public's knowledge about AIDS and sexual practices. Simultaneously, a press conference was organized to dispel misconceptions about AIDS transmission and prevention. The results of the second survey revealed gaps in knowledge that needed to be filled.

We then elaborated a systematic educational programme for AIDS prevention. It was at that point, in selecting the contents of the educational material, that we experienced some difficulty with the Roman Catholic Church. The Church was concerned about the references to the use of condoms in the educational material. It also considered all homosexual and bisexual men to be sinners and was opposed to giving them any assistance. To cope with this very difficult situation we met the Archbishop many times to discuss ethical and moral values and to review the educational material produced. Finally the church agreed to work with infected patients and to disseminate information about AIDS to poor people living in the slums. Today its attitude has changed to such an extent that it says we are not doing enough. It has stopped objecting to the use of condoms.

Our AIDS prevention programme was launched in February 1986. The television spots, lasting 30 seconds to one minute, showed: the safety of blood donation under specified conditions; compassion towards the AIDS patient; the use of condoms as a safe means of avoiding AIDS; mechanisms of transmission; mechanisms of non-transmission; and AIDS and drugs. The printed media – newspapers and magazines – reinforced the messages. At the same time radio messages were broadcast through 6000 radio stations for three consecutive months.

To develop the public's awareness of the danger of AIDS, the Ministry of Health also published a pamphlet on AIDS, which it inserted in the monthly electricity and water bills, and the pay cheques of employees of ministries, private enterprises, and nongovernmental organizations. In addition, during the carnival, a time of greater sexual permissiveness, the Ministry of Health published a pamphlet in four languages; it was distributed at the country's main ports of entry and warned travellers of the risk of contracting AIDS through casual sexual encounters, intravenous drug abuse, and blood transfusions. The pamphlet also recommended the use of condoms during sexual intercourse.

Groups engaging in high-risk behaviour

The high-risk groups consist of homosexual and bisexual men, intravenous drug users, and male and female prostitutes. Haemophiliacs specifically requested that no educational materials or TV messages should be aimed at them as a group. They do not consider themselves as engaging in dangerous behaviour since they are the unwilling victims of infected blood and blood products.

Television items on high-risk behaviour were broadcast late at night to enable speakers to talk openly and objectively about sex. Leaflets on the same subject were published. Evaluation indicated that the most receptive target audiences were homosexual and bisexual men and teenagers, and that they had changed their sexual behaviour to a noticeable extent.

Adolescents

Adolescents we consider to be the most vulnerable group. The result of the lack of sex education in schools and homes is that 33% of all pregnancies and 26% of all abortions occur among teenagers and they show a high incidence of sexually transmitted diseases in both urban and rural areas. In rural areas people live closely together with little or no privacy, and this stimulates promiscuity and early sexual activity and often the multiplication of large families in poor health.

The young are exposed to the erotic influence of the media, which encourages them to experiment with sex while they are still unprepared for it. To cope with this problem the Ministers of Health and of Education are taking joint action to reduce the incidence of sexually transmitted diseases, including AIDS, and to teach sex as an expression of life. The action includes the training of teachers and the preparation of sex education/STD/AIDS manuals.

Conclusion

What lessons have we drawn from our initial programme?

It was a positive experience to have diverse segments of society represented in the elaboration of the education programme, such as the

Roman Catholic Church and homosexual groups. This collaboration was sometimes stressful, but it created conditions for designing a programme that is acceptable to a great variety of audiences. Several messages were recognized as outstanding:

- the slogan "Love does not kill"
- a television broadcast on compassion for AIDS patients presented by the actress, Irene Ravache
- a television broadcast on sex and AIDS
- a television broadcast on AIDS and intravenous drug users.

A negative experience was the censuring of many television broadcasts by the Ministry of Health and the Roman Catholic Church and the cutback in funds, which hampered the effectiveness of the media.

On the basis of our evaluation we would, on the whole, maintain the same content and strategies, but consider the following changes:

(1) more reliance on the private sector for the financing and implementation of the programme; and
(2) different ways of approaching prostitutes and intravenous drug users, the two groups for which the programme proved ineffective in changing attitudes towards AIDS prevention.

Preventing AIDS Through General Public Education: Experience from the United Kingdom

SPENCER HAGARD

Dr Spencer Hagard is Director of the Health Education Authority, London. Striking aspects of the United Kingdom AIDS education programme have been the very strong government leadership and constructive partnership of the normally competitive mass media.

By the end of 1987, 1227 cases of AIDS had been reported in the United Kingdom, with 697 deaths. The great majority of our AIDS cases (84%) arose from male homosexual or bisexual transmission. Significant minorities were recipients of infected blood or blood products, people infected through heterosexual intercourse, intravenous drug users, and children born of infected mothers.

The United Kingdom public health strategy to combat AIDS has three main components:

- services for people with AIDS and HIV infection
- specific measures to control the spread of infection (e.g., screening of blood, tissue, and organ donors)
- public health education aimed at the general public as well as at people at particular risk.

Educating the general public

Early in 1986 the United Kingdom Department of Health and the Central Office of Information commissioned a nationwide mass media campaign with the aim of:

- educating people about the facts of AIDS
- dispelling myths
- offering appropriate advice and reassurance
- influencing social opinion so as to change attitudes and modify risk behaviour in the long term.

The campaign was pragmatic rather than moralizing in tone, in the expectation that that would be more likely to be effective.

General newspaper advertising started during March 1986 and continued through the next eight months, with feedback and evaluation. This was followed by a concerted campaign of posters, radio, and television. In January 1987 a leaflet was distributed to all 25 million households in the United Kingdom. At the same time, thanks to impressive media cooperation, there was extensive television, radio, and newspaper coverage, with special programmes and features, culminating in an "AIDS Week on TV" during February 1987 when at least 35 AIDS-related programmes were screened during 19 hours of programming. This was supported by a national telephone information, advice, and leaflet-ordering service.

In September 1987 the second stage of the campaign was aimed at drug users, discouraging in particular drug use by injection and the sharing of equipment.

Additional provision has been made for supplying information to the blind and deaf and to people whose first language is not English.

The mass media campaign has been well supported by intersectoral initiatives involving national and local government authorities and voluntary agencies.

Evaluation of the mass media campaign

Evaluation of the campaign was seen to be very important, its main results being as follows. Very few people amongst those questioned found the advertising offensive and nearly all adults agreed that it was right for the Government to undertake such a campaign. Awareness of the information provided by the media, though quite high before the campaign, reached the extremely high figure of 96% amongst those questioned. It is estimated that three-quarters of adults had read or looked through the leaflet distributed to all households. All this helped to create an atmosphere in our society in which AIDS could be discussed.

Amongst those questioned, knowledge about how AIDS is transmitted was high before the campaign but increased further, particularly knowledge about heterosexual intercourse and needle-sharing. The usefulness of condoms as a protective measure was also understood. There is also evidence of reduction in myths and misconceptions, with one important exception: 39% of people in February 1987 believed that AIDS could be acquired by donating blood. No significant self-reported change, however, had occurred in heterosexual behaviour. This was not unexpected at that stage of the campaign.

With regard to homosexuals, their knowledge and awareness was already very high even before the media campaign. This is attributable to several years of health education by national and local voluntary organizations. Looking for evidence of changes in homosexual behaviour, we found a reduction in risky sexual behaviour and in the numbers of sexual partners. This change has been sustained, as illustrated by data showing a reduction in other sexually transmitted diseases amongst homosexuals.

Conclusion

I should like to emphasize the key points from the experience of the United Kingdom. These are:

(1) Government leadership, which acted as a catalyst in achieving public acceptability.
(2) The importance of pre-planning, with clear objective-setting and inbuilt monitoring and evaluation. This enables the best use to be made of limited resources.
(3) A constructive partnership amongst the normally very competitive mass media (with corresponding coverage gained on radio and television and in the popular press).
(4) Positive collateral effects on policy and practice in such fields as employment, housing, and education.
(5) The greater effectiveness of a national campaign if it is strongly linked to local needs, wants, and activities. This linkage has yet to be fully developed in the United Kingdom. It should be emphasized that the campaign is dynamic, evolving as public needs change.

In conclusion, our future needs in the United Kingdom are to maintain awareness and encourage and sustain prudent behaviour. The challenge is how to do this positively and constructively within the overall national policy of promoting health for all.

PART III

Theory into Practice: Health Promotion Programmes for Specific Groups

This part of the proceedings shows that programmes and strategies can be designed for and aimed at particular target audiences. The examples given are:

- women in New York City
- adolescents in Denmark
- aboriginal and islander communities in Australia
- women prostitutes in Nairobi
- homosexual men in Switzerland.

Dr Jake Obetsebe-Lamptey, who has extensive experience, mainly in Africa, of social marketing and professional advertising in health promotion campaigns, introduces the subject. He stresses the importance of motivating vulnerable groups to accept responsibility for protecting themselves against HIV infection.

Introduction

JAKE OBETSEBE-LAMPTEY*

As regards the child and her parents described by Dr Meyer (page 23), this Summit may be too late. They were infected with AIDS in the night of our ignorance. They did not know. We did not know. It is now morning and we are awake. We can have no excuse for permitting others to become infected because of ignorance about AIDS. We may not yet have a vaccine or a cure for AIDS, but we can teach people the facts and give them the reasons to change high-risk behaviour and the support to sustain the change over time.

We address ourselves today to the future, to intervening now to prevent tomorrow's catastrophe, because we can, we must, we will make a difference.

Dr Jonathan Mann presented us with a challenge. To prevent the spread of AIDS, he said we must seek to influence positively the behaviour of individuals and groups with our most effective strategies. If AIDS had to come, then it has come into a world which can fight back, a world which is armed with a tested communication capability that has already been proven in other public health challenges such as the prevention of heart disease and smoking, oral rehydration therapy, immunization, and family planning.

For effective use of this capability, which exists in every country, many of us must put aside our prejudices; we must change some of our attitudes so that we can communicate and stop merely lecturing. We hope to show how the real involvement of the people one is communicating with leads to meaningful education and moves away from "we know what is best for you". We also hope to show that, as AIDS affects us all, so too all must be allowed to participate in its prevention. We must lose the prejudices that hamper us from using the total arsenal at our disposal, be it private or public, paid for or voluntary, formal or informal. It is true that the government cannot do this alone; the government needs outside skills, institutional networks. But it is also very true that without government support no private initiative can long succeed.

* Managing Director, Lintas Worldwide (Educational Programmes), Ghana.

The challenge is to influence positively the behaviour of individuals and groups with our most effective strategies. WHO staff members said that they are confident that people who have learned and wish to use what they have learned, who are influenced positively by others, and who have the opportunity and support to modify their behaviour will do so. This confidence would seem to be well placed. The evidence is already coming in, from San Francisco and Zurich, from Nairobi, that those who have learned, who have wished to use what they have learned, who have been supported positively by their peers, and who have had the opportunity are modifying their behaviour. Here is where we find encouragement that our work as communicators will make a difference. Here also is where we find the lessons that will help us to make the difference in the future.

Examples of four broad national strategies have been given. These national strategies are like a giant umbrella, sheltering dozens of specific private and public activities addressed to specific audiences – men who have sex with men, schoolchildren, intravenous drug users, women, persons with haemophilia, prostitutes, opinion leaders, health workers, club owners, and so on. Together these activities create a whole greater than the simple sum of its parts. These intensive efforts targeted at specific populations and emerging from their values are providing the support people need to change high-risk behaviour.

The following papers from Australia, Denmark, Kenya, the Netherlands, Switzerland, and the United States, deal with just one aspect of their programmes. We recognize that their programmes are more comprehensive and complex than they will have time to explain, but concentration on a single aspect illustrates the importance of the communication process in successful AIDS health promotion, as seen in terms of planning, implementation, monitoring, and evaluation.

Planning

The first element in planning is to learn about the disease and the behaviour of people in relation to it so that we can define our target audience. While we are all affected by this disease, some people, because of their behaviour, are at higher risk. It is risk behaviour and not class of people that helps us to define our target audience. The example of New York City illustrates the targeting of audiences on the basis of behaviour. The New York City example is about women. While we were preparing for this meeting someone asked: "Supposing a Summit participant asks the question 'Why women? After all, what percentage of AIDS sufferers in New York can be women?' " The answer was "That was a good question five years ago, but today AIDS is the biggest single cause of death of women in New York between the ages 25 and 34." There are countries that do not yet have an AIDS problem. Let us hope that they will not have the same question to answer five years from now.

Implementation

Once we have a target group we must learn from them what they already know about AIDS, their attitudes towards AIDS, towards health, towards risk, their full range of practices and how ingrained they are, how susceptible they are to change. The paper on the Danish adolescents and school programme shows that we should not assume that we know the answers, that we must work with our audience to get the information we need from them. It shows the dangers for communicators in making assumptions. Far too often our assumptions are based on simplistic stereotypes.

The paper on the Australian aboriginal and islander people highlights development of the message. In the paper we are taken into a process that is as old as time, the process called "consultation". The paper demonstrates the role of the target audience in creating the message – a role that can be played by that audience only – and shows how we must involve our audience if we are to communicate effectively.

A message, however good, that is not seen or heard cannot communicate. While some of our target audiences can be reached easily, others for a variety of reasons are far more difficult to reach. However, as the papers from Kenya and the Netherlands show, by using the existing infrastructure, skills available in the community, creativity, members of the target audience, persistence, and repetition of the message, even the most hard to reach can be reached.

Monitoring and evaluation

The final element in the process is monitoring and evaluation. Programmes need to be monitored and evaluated to provide the necessary direction for growth and change, to help to right what is wrong and to do better what is right. Monitoring and evaluation start at the planning stage, where we set measurable objectives, and continue throughout all aspects of implementation. As the paper from Switzerland shows, monitoring and evaluation are not always formal and structured activities. They are ongoing and may involve bar-room conversation as much as studies focused on groups, anecdotes as much as surveys. They must be ongoing; they cannot be deferred for lack of time, effort, finance, or other reasons. We all make mistakes; the bad mistakes we make are those we leave uncorrected and those we do not learn from.

I repeat – we want people who engage in high-risk behaviour to change what they do. We want people to take action to protect themselves from HIV infection. The whole process of effective communication recognizes the differences in people, in situations, in cultures, in mores. The papers that follow are examples of what has been done to illustrate the process of how to communicate effectively and motivate people to act.

Health promotion will be effective only if the process of planning, implementation, monitoring, and evaluation is correctly employed in accordance with needs and resources.

Messages Addressed to Women as a Target Audience

PEGGY CLARKE

Ms Peggy Clarke is Assistant Commissioner for AIDS Program Training, New York City. She describes a media-based health education component of an AIDS control programme directed particularly at women, which helps dispel the notion that AIDS is a disease of homosexual men only.

In the United States of America, where the number of AIDS cases exceeds 50000, many people are under the mistaken impression that AIDS is a disease of homosexual men, a gay disease. To communicate AIDS prevention messages to people at risk, we must shatter this myth and tailor prevention programmes to others at risk who are not homosexual men. Women are just such an audience. New York City has over 12000 people with AIDS, of whom 10% are females. AIDS is the leading cause of death in women aged 25–34 in New York City.

The risk behaviour of women with AIDS is primarily intravenous drug use, or being the sexual partner of an intravenous drug user or a bisexual man. Women who have AIDS are only a small proportion of those who are at risk from their sexual or drug behaviour. For our programme to be effective, women must learn that AIDS is not only a gay disease but one that may affect them as well.

Numerous polls and surveys have indicated that knowledge about AIDS is very high in the United States. However, the extent of change to lower-risk behaviour does not correspond with the level of knowledge. Our task is to bridge the gap between what people *know* and what they *do* to protect themselves.

In our media planning we target women as a special audience. However, women are not all alike; they vary greatly in their perception of their own risk of contracting AIDS. This variability reflects their diverse social, cultural, and ethnic backgrounds as well as the responsibilities and roles they assume in their lives. These different roles have shaped and directed our campaign.

We narrowed down the different audiences of women we wanted to reach and designed specific messages for each one. Our analysis was

51

based on academic research, field observations, and interviews with women in different situations throughout the city. The advertising industry regularly shapes messages to appeal to different audiences in order to sell products. We utilized the same techniques in these campaigns to sell AIDS prevention. We organized four different television campaigns, targeted at adolescent women, women as parents, sexually active women, and women who have sex with partners in long-term relationships. Each campaign uses a particular approach to appeal to a particular audience and describes the action that is being promoted as the means of preventing transmission. Each has a companion strategy for radio and printed matter.

In the first campaign a young woman with AIDS expresses her regret at having become pregnant at an early age and given birth to a child with AIDS. The message here promotes the idea of sexual abstinence, a rather unpopular concept on American television. Using a teenage girl to tell her story acknowledges the strong influence peer groups have on young people and strengthens the credibility of the message.

The second message, which depicts a mother talking openly to her child, is aimed at parents who may want to ignore the issue of AIDS or be inclined to leave the responsibility for educating their children to teachers, the media, or the children's peers. Here we ask parents to put aside their embarrassment and their fear of encouraging sex and talk about AIDS before it hits home. The aim is to stimulate discussion between parents and children and to demonstrate one method of talking openly about AIDS prevention. In the Spanish adaptation the mother's embarrassment is more apparent, reflecting different cultural mores in the Hispanic community in New York City.

Two messages are addressed to sexually active women. The first depicts a young woman who is preparing for a date and whose preparation includes placing a condom in her handbag. It challenges all sexually active women not to deny the risk of AIDS. This is a woman who is thinking ahead and, by accepting responsibility for self-protection, is in control of her own life. The companion printed text advises "Don't Go Out Without Your Rubbers". The second message shows a couple on the verge of intimate sexual relations. The woman offers the man a condom, and he rejects it; she departs. This message suggests that a sexually active woman should negotiate the terms of a relationship before sexual intimacy begins. She then maintains the ability to remove herself from a risky situation.

For the fourth group, women in long-term relationships, the spot begins with the death of a baby from AIDS and follows with a flashback showing the father contracting the virus from intravenous drug use and passing it to his wife through sexual intercourse. The message here is that recognition of risk behaviour is essential, even in a long-standing and continuing relationship, to ensure that preventive action can be taken. Because of the strong link between intravenous drug use and heterosexual transmission, this campaign message is especially important for women in New York City.

The primary message in all of these campaigns is that communication in relationships is a critical component of AIDS prevention. However, because women are in different relationships and have different responsibilities, the campaigns must differ in order to reach different female populations directly.

The media can play a significant role in changing cultural norms within a society and in fostering open discussion of formerly taboo topics. These campaigns have greatly magnified the visibility of the AIDS issue for women in New York City. We have witnessed changes in the content of movies, plays, television shows, and song lyrics, changes that reflect a greater awareness of AIDS and the risk of heterosexual transmission.

Finally, it is important to remember that media-based health education is only a small part of the comprehensive effort to combat this epidemic. Research, expanded voluntary counselling, HIV testing, condom distribution, and school health promotion along with responsible legislative action and increased drug addiction services are all fundamental to effective action for the elimination of AIDS as a threat to the public health.

Adolescents: Knowledge, Attitudes and Practice

LONE DE NEERGAARD

Dr Lone de Neergaard is AIDS coordinator at the National Board of Health, Copenhagen, Denmark. She describes an intensive programme focused on adolescents, which involves them in preparing materials, uses humour and explicit pictures, and draws on public figures, with a view to promoting responsible sexual behaviour and respect for the positive aspects of sex.

We can learn a lot from one another, but the information to be transmitted in each country has to be adjusted to the particular country at the particular time. Although we can get ideas from others, programmes must be developed with due respect for our own traditions and culture.

You may know Denmark as a country with a so-called free-sex morality. Some may like this, some may not, but it has been an advantage to us in our battle against AIDS; it makes it much easier to talk about AIDS when you call things by their common names and even show explicit pictures. Denmark may be unique in this respect, and I therefore ask you to view my account not as an example of how things should be done but rather of how things are being done in Denmark.

Why is it important to focus on adolescents?

Focus on adolescents is important for three reasons:

(1) They are in the process of forming habits and can thus be influenced.
(2) They will go through a period with changing partners and hence are at risk.
(3) By learning at an early age future problems will be prevented, and it is therefore a good investment to start early.

Why knowledge, attitudes, and practice?

It is not enough for adolescents to know the facts about AIDS; they also have to be motivated to apply the knowledge when it matters. This applies particularly to sexual practices. Many other factors influence young people; many other messages come into their minds. One of the characteristics of adolescents is to rebel against the right, the sensible, the recommendable thing to do. Sometimes they may even embark upon risk behaviour for the fun of it. Altogether, communicating with adolescents about AIDS can be difficult.

We are not sure that we can achieve a permanent change in young people's behaviour by using fear. We use humour instead. In spite of the seriousness of the problem we find humour a good opener to young people's minds.

Methods of study

We studied sexual knowledge, attitudes, and practices among adolescents in several ways. Since we were dealing with very private topics we had to avoid traditional methods and develop new ones. We inquire about young people's knowledge and attitudes at the same time as we give them new information. One method, which produced many fascinating results, was an essay competition, for which all schoolchildren aged 14–15 years in Copenhagen were asked to write on their thoughts about AIDS. This is one of the many ways in which young people can learn and at the same time express their feelings about this new threat to their world.

Of course, the results of such inquiries are derived from reports on one's own behaviour. Only figures for the spread of HIV or for the numbers of sexually transmitted diseases tell us exactly about the effects of changing practices. Nevertheless, we do get from self-reports very useful information about trends, and by repeating the surveys over time we can follow their development.

Our results show that there are many myths about sex and AIDS. In one school class 15-year-old students said that they had 15-20 partners, mostly using safe sex. When we asked about the price of a condom there was deep silence. We guessed that the silence reflected more of the truth than the claim of safe sex. We also found that such aspects as negative discrimination, minority groups, and how to deal with HIV-positive people were much more a concern of young people than we had expected. We found that young people are generally very tolerant.

Messages and channels

We used the results of our inquiries to devise means of filling the gaps we had discovered in knowledge and attitudes.

Knowledge

The extent of the knowledge of the young is considerable. Our main tasks are to maintain and increase their awareness and to ensure they obtain a realistic understanding of the risk to themselves.

What we did was to create an advertisement with questions and answers composed by ourselves. It was published in the main newspapers and in weekly and monthly journals for adolescents. It was very well received. It was also easy to produce, which meant that we were able to correct misunderstandings in the media soon after they occurred.

Attitudes

Attitudes towards AIDS are very polarized; they are typically either the "not-me" syndrome or the "everyone is going to die of AIDS" fear. Our main focus is to stress:

- one has personal responsibility for oneself
- sex is good and healthy
- condoms must be demystified, made commonly known, accepted
- safe sex is essential; everybody has the same problem
- discrimination is not justified, neither are negative reactions to HIV-positive people
- AIDS concerns you and me and everybody else.

To make this message effective we asked more than 200 well-known Danes to participate in our new television and radio campaign for young people. Politicians, administrators, actors, football players and many others now come together in 22 television spots. A poster brings all this together under the slogan "Think twice". As a consequence to media coverage of English football players not being allowed to hug and kiss after a match, we put this advertisement in the sporting sections of the big newspapers. The message was effective.

To transmit the message "Sex is good and healthy and beautiful, and we want it to stay that way", we had advertisements and a poster printed. The poster became very popular and is now found in many young people's rooms.

To make condoms less mysterious and widely known and accepted, we designed six-metre-long posters for the sides of buses, showing condoms, with the text: "Protect the one you love". It certainly attracted attention, and although we were critized for focusing too much on safe sex we had very few negative reactions. The message was printed in six different languages, not for tourists but to attract the attention of the Danes.

Practice

We want young people to change the way they practise sex; we do not expect them to abandon sex altogether. We found that explicit information in the form of pictures, cartoons, and videos was necessary in order to show exactly what safe sex is.

Pamphlets showing how to use condoms were distributed to supermarkets, petrol stations, kiosks, pharmacies, etc.

Main tactics

The main principles or rules that guide our AIDS information programme for adolescents are:

- make such education life-oriented, not death-directed
- minimize fear
- minimize discrimination
- integrate information with other sex and health education (we know that the need for AIDS information makes sex education more acceptable than before)
- make education open and direct
- include face-to-face communication (pamphlets and posters go only part of the way)
- make education multisectoral – in schools, clubs, sports, the arts, etc.
- make education practical – talk about, show, buy, try condoms
- make sure condoms are easily available
- make safe sex smart, "in", the status thing.

It is our experience that by far the best way to develop materials is by working together with the young or by letting them do it themselves. We have produced plenty of good material, some of which the young found too boring or just not what they wanted to do. It is amazing to see the creativity of a group of young people who want to do something about AIDS.

Generally, teachers have cooperated very well and have accepted the need for the information; indeed, many teachers themselves began to teach about AIDS very early on. Of course, some found it difficult to embark on discussions about sex, and this must be respected. From the practical point of view, teachers are not good educators if they do not feel comfortable with a topic.

We still have many unanswered questions about AIDS prevention, and new questions arise every day. However, one thing is now clear: we must act now to protect our adolescent population from infection, even if the number of HIV infections among adolescents is low. Four to five years ago we made the mistake of believing that AIDS affected only homosexuals. Today we see women and children die as the disease spreads to all our people. We must not make this mistake again. If we are lucky and the infection does not spread as we fear, and if the numbers stay low over the next two to three years, then I shall be pleased to admit that I was wrong, that we did not need to do all we are doing today. However, if the disease spreads, as we expect it will, in no way shall I be prepared to commit the same mistake as we made before – to underestimate the threat and allow thousands more to die.

Developing Materials for Culture Groups

GRACE SMALLWOOD

Ms Grace Smallwood is a community health worker and health educator in an AIDS control programme for aborigines at Townsville, Queensland, Australia, and a member of the Australian National Advisory Council on AIDS.

Condoms or quandongs? A small lapse in communication illustrates the problems of adapting educating activities to cultural characteristics and involving communities actively in health promotion.

I want to talk about an approach to developing media and educational AIDS materials for a specific culture, which is applicable to societies that have limited technical, professional, and monetary resources. This is not a top-down approach but one that uses aboriginal and islander health workers as the key people in the conception, development, and implementation of AIDS education programmes.

Many aboriginal/islander people in Australia have a health status similar to that of people in Third World countries. There is a high prevalence of drug abuse, widespread malnutrition, a poor living environment, inadequate essential services, a low educational achievement, and high unemployment. To overcome these problems requires collaboration and consultation with aboriginal/islander communities, which form an integral part of our cultural heritage spanning over 40000 years.

The approach taken to AIDS education in aboriginal/islander communities has three main components:

- *consultation*, taking place *in* aboriginal/islander communities with local people
- *networking*, using established aboriginal/islander health worker networks
- *pre-testing of communication materials*, which involves aboriginal/islander health workers in developing, pre-testing, and running public health campaigns.

The reasons for working with aboriginal/islander health workers are that they have:

- a practical knowledge of their culture
- a commitment to raising the health status of the community
- a knowledge of local health issues
- an understanding of the difficulties facing the resolution of any problem in the community
- a degree of recognition in the community that visiting experts cannot quickly achieve.

Our programme is based on a series of workshops. It is essential that the workshops take place in aboriginal/islander communities, so that opinions are heard in the most natural and realistic setting. It is also important to gain the cooperation of workshop participants quickly so that they will freely contribute their ideas.

The workshop team consists of a doctor, a nurse, a health educator, a communication consultant, and a graphic artist. Two of these people are aborigines or islanders.

The workshop begins with short introductions and information sessions about AIDS. They are followed by sessions on basic rules of communication, how to develop media materials, and how to plan a health education campaign. Deciding on aims and objectives, selecting target audiences, and developing messages to be conveyed are key elements of this process. The ideas of the workshop participants are recorded and the graphic artist and communication consultant develop several concepts based on them. On the following day the concepts are presented in rough visual form to the workshop. The participants are enthusiastic in their response when they see their ideas expressed visually. Once again note is taken of the participants' reactions to the various concepts, particularly what people say, how they react – with laughter, puzzlement, seriousness – and, most important, their ideas for changes. These changes are then incorporated into further versions of the materials.

Community members are then invited to view and comment on the materials so as to obtain a wider audience response and refine the materials to a final acceptable stage. The workshop then determines which posters, slogans, or advertisements it thinks are the strongest and most effective.

The next session of the workshop develops action plans on specific activities that can be undertaken in the campaign. The action plans bring together networking, research, planning, and evaluation. These elements are then developed into specific activities related to the networks used by health workers.

Thus the materials go through several stages to reach the final product. To illustrate this process, I shall tell you the story of "condoman". The term "condoman" was developed to counteract the embarrassment, or "shame" as we call it, caused by the use of condoms. In my community condoms are known as "frenchies", and from my own experience I can tell you a story that highlights the need to use the local language when talking about AIDS. I was talking to a group of local women about the need to use condoms to prevent AIDS and, because the use of condoms was regarded as shameful, I kept stressing the need for it. Later that night one of the women telephoned me to say she did not know why I was so worried about AIDS, because they had plenty of quandong trees in their area. I suddenly realized that she had confused "condom" with a local tree called a "quandong" and thought that AIDS could be prevented by eating quandong fruit. So, in this locality, people had to be persuaded to overcome their shame and be prepared to use condoms; but condoms also had to be called "frenchies" so that people would not confuse them with fruit trees!

Just a final point. We have used the colours red, yellow, and black, because they are the colours of the aboriginal flag and are instantly recognizable by aboriginal/islander people. This is another example of being culturally specific in communication. When aboriginal people see these colours they know that the communication is for them and they trust the message.

The most important aspect of the training workshop is that it produces materials – posters, radio advertisements, action plans – on the spot and pre-tests them in local communities. This approach reinforces the importance of aboriginal/islander health workers and develops strategies that fit into existing structures and networks. It also trains health workers in the essential process of conceiving, planning, and implementing a media campaign concerned with health issues. Most important, the health education programme that is developed is relevant to the particular community and is "owned" by the community.

AIDS Prevention in the Netherlands: Intravenous Drug Users as a Target Group

HANS MOERKERK

Dr Hans Moerkerk, of the Netherlands, a political scientist and psychologist, is Director of the Health Education Centre, Amsterdam, Secretary of the National AIDS Commission of the Netherlands, and member of the Expert Committee on AIDS of the Council of Europe. In Amsterdam, long experience of unconventional forms of health care for intravenous drug users has helped in incorporating new AIDS prevention strategies into municipal programmes, with the cooperation of drug users, and health care and social workers.

It is noon on a normal working-day in Amsterdam, the old capital of the Kingdom of the Netherlands. A rebuilt city bus is leaving its garage to perform its daily duty as a mobile outdoor clinic for drug users, who receive their daily dose of methadone, personal counselling, free condoms, and a new supply of clean syringes and needles in exchange for used ones. Since 1985 three of these vehicles have been used for this purpose in association with several centres at fixed addresses. Like so many other cities in the world, Amsterdam has such problems as unemployment, a high crime rate, housing shortages, and drug abuse. Amsterdam is also an attractive town, popular with tourists and also with young people, who try to live their own way of life there.

Since 1975 the municipal government has developed a number of programmes focused on health care for drug addicts, sometimes by very unconventional methods. Although the use of hard drugs is illegal, we have learned to accept the use of drugs as a reality in society. Since AIDS has developed in our country, this attitude proved to be effective in the fight against the disease. This small country of 14 million inhabitants has 420 registered cases of AIDS; 16 of them are intravenous drug users, mostly of heroin. The vast majority live in Amsterdam; many of them come from abroad.

In 1983 the municipal health service started an integrated drug programme which was accepted by the city council. This programme provides for better cooperation between the police, health care facilities, and the municipal authorities. The national Government has supported the programme politically and financially. The programme has four objectives:

(1) Contact.
(2) Harm reduction.
(3) Drug-free treatment.
(4) Resocialization.

Contact

Street-corner workers, doctors, and specialized social psychiatric nurses have access to places where concentrations of addicts are found. These places include police stations, in which we are able to meet an increasing number of addicts (2500 in 1987), and general hospitals, where we can visit an increasing number of addicts also (400 in 1987).

Regular contact with addicts is a necessary condition for preventive action. Daily experience with addicts teaches us to be realistic; most are caught within a pattern of drug use, rehabilitation, and relapse.

Harm reduction

In our experience harm reduction is the second best aim if it is not possible to cure the addict. It involves extensive medical and social care, methadone distribution, and needle exchange. Methadone distribution is seen as a major way of reducing harm. It is used as a means of establishing an arrangement with drug addicts that provides them with the best medical and social care and gives them a starting-point in stabilization of the addiction. Participation in the methadone programme is increasing rapidly; in 1987, 5000 addicts took part in it, or about 75% of the drug-addicted population.

At present 4.5% of the AIDS cases in Holland are intravenous drug users. This is still a small number, but studies among this group indicate an HIV seropositivity rate of 30%. Because of frequent needle-sharing and sexual contacts, for example in prostitution, intravenous drug users can transmit the virus to other larger groups of the population. It is therefore essential to organize an infrastructure of harm-reduction facilities where contact with intravenous drug addicts can easily be made. The method we have been using since 1985 aims at behaviour change, which can be achieved only if certain conditions are fulfilled:

(1) There must be a continuous provision of information about safe use and safe sex. Personal contact is the best way of bringing the message to the addicts.
(2) Condoms must be distributed free of charge in many places to facilitate safe sex.

(3) There must be easy access to health care facilities for medical care, for counselling to support drug-free treatment, and for methadone distribution.

Amsterdam has various methadone projects at different levels. The most obvious is the 'methadone by bus' project, but there are also outpatient methadone clinics as well as general practitioners who take part in the project. As most of the addicts visit the facilities frequently, they are used for the exchange of needles and syringes.

The needle and syringe exchange scheme began in the summer of 1984. AIDS and the spread of hepatitis B inspired the so-called Junky Union, a league of drug addicts that proposed the exchange programme, which was already under preparation. The municipal health service supported them in an experimental scheme in 1984 and it has been established since 1985. It expanded rapidly, with more than 700000 exchanges in 1987. The expansion was accompanied by a considerable decrease in the numbers of needle-sharing addicts, from 75% in 1985 to only 25% in 1987. Of course we were aware of the disadvantages and possible criticisms of the scheme – were we encouraging drug abuse, and would there be a black market in needles, which would be sold for money to buy illegal drugs?

The scheme had clear advantages, however: intravenous drug users would reduce needle-sharing and this could slow down substantially the spread of HIV; and they would pay more attention to better hygiene, be more accessible to AIDS information, and refrain from injecting themselves with used syringes and needles.

The municipality as well as the Government decided to make this model a part of the national strategy in the fight against AIDS, since the early findings gave an indication of positive results.

Summary of AIDS prevention policy in the Netherlands since 1983

1. Preventive activities were aimed first at people at greatest risk of HIV infection: men who have sex with men and intravenous drug users. More groups were, and will be, incorporated, such as prostitutes and their customers, adolescents, tourists, migrant workers, and professional groups. These preventive activities are being built up by a step-by-step approach.

2. It is essential to distinguish between health information and health education. People first need information, the facts, as the essential foundation for the second step, health education for those who need to change their behaviour, to protect themselves and others from HIV infection. Health education means much more than giving people the necessary information, and it does not use fear as a means of changing

their behaviour since undue fear would lead them to ignore the message.

3. Although nationwide information campaigns were organized, priority has been given to programmes directed at specific target groups. A variety of educational activities have been organized for them.

4. Prevention policy in the Netherlands aims at maximum effectiveness.

5. The programme is differentiated and target-group-specific.

6. There is permanent monitoring of the input and impact of the programme, to ensure the rationality of the measures.

7. The continuity and consistency of the programme are considered to have the maximum priority.

8. According to the recommendations of the European Economic Community, the Council of Europe, and WHO, we try to keep our activities free of secondary aims and value judgements.

9 We consider it essential to include everybody involved in AIDS in the organization of the prevention programme. Consensus gives maximum effectiveness.

To coordinate and organize all the activities undertaken, the National Task Force in AIDS has been accorded official status by the Secretary of State for Health and, even more important, a government-controlled budget, that can be used for prevention, care, and research.

AIDS needs an integrated policy, not only on a national scale but also at the international level. To make a worldwide effort possible, the Netherlands is therefore also active in international bodies such as WHO, the European Economic Community, and the Council of Europe.

Reaching the Target Population: Female Prostitutes

ELIZABETH NGUGI

Mrs Elizabeth Njeri Ngugi, a registered nurse from Kenya, is chairwoman of the Health Education Committee of Kenya's National AIDS Committee and Lecturer, Department of Community Health, University of Nairobi. She describes here how a study group worked with a large group of prostitutes to bring about a dramatic increase in the proportion of prostitutes insisting on the use of condoms and a demand for rehabilitation.

Allow me to make an obvious statement: prostitutes are human beings. They want to belong and to be appreciated. They want to be involved in their own wellbeing. Like other people, they want the best for their children. They are glad and proud when we invite them to become partners in curbing the spread of the HIV virus. They bring a wealth of useful practical knowledge to this partnership.

Monogamy with uninfected partners is the least-risk type of sexual relationship. However, not everybody follows this lifestyle. Prostitutes are usually unable or unwilling to find other occupations. Nor, often, are their clients able or willing to find other sexual outlets. Then the condom serves as prophylaxis against the AIDS virus, just as chloroquine protects against malaria.

Prostitutes are normally a hard-to-reach group (their clients are even harder to reach). We walked in the mud, in the rain, and in the sun in our effort to meet these women where they live and work, in order to establish a rapport with them and gain their trust and confidence. We approached them as we would any other group of women. We did not call them prostitutes. *They* told us who they were.

After much effort we were able to bring about 300 of these women together at a *baraza* (public meeting). They told us what their needs were in the control and prevention of sexually transmitted diseases. We had no cases of AIDS in Kenya at that time. We explained to them how infection is transmitted and what its effects are. We told them how infection can be prevented. We invited them to register at a new clinic that was established specifically to serve them. Eventually over 700 women registered. In their enthusiasm for protecting their own health they elected a leader and a committee to represent the three urban communities where they lived.

We trained the committee members in community mobilization and basic communication skills, in order to promote the use of condoms. They acted as informal health educators of the others. We told them that HIV detection and surveillance were to commence. We invited all the women to take part. The committee met the health team every two months, and *barazas* took place every six months.

At one of these *barazas* with about 300 women present, we told them that our HIV studies showed that some of them were infected with the AIDS virus and other sexually transmitted infections. We explained that those who were infected were likely to transmit the infection to their clients, and that those who were not infected were at risk of becoming infected. The best thing they could do, we told them, was to cease prostitution, the next best to insist that their clients use condoms.

We used several educational methods. The first was a written test of the women's knowledge of AIDS, of their ability to prevent it, and of how they would teach others to prevent getting AIDS. About 250 women took the test. The 10 with the best answers were invited to address a gathering of the other women. They shared with them their knowledge and skills, and impressed upon them the nature and the consequences of infection with the virus. The second method was skits and role-playing. The members of the committee acted in them to reinforce the earlier messages. The third method was a song to be sung by members of the committee at a *baraza*. The fourth method was group and individual counselling, to enable the women and ourselves to discuss their problems and how best to solve them.

One thing that came out during counselling was that most of the women would like to change their lifestyle, to give up prostitution. They asked for a rehabilitation programme to retrain them for other suitable work, as a starting-point for a new life.

The result of these joint efforts was a dramatic increase in condom use. At the beginning 8% of the women insisted occasionally that their clients use condoms. After a year more than 50% were making their clients use condoms all the time, and a further 40% did so occasionally. We believe that the figures are now even higher. These changes, arising from such a modest educational input, were truly remarkable; as you may know, condoms are not readily accepted as a method of contraception in Africa.

The outcome of all this was a threefold reduction in the rate of seroconversion from HIV-negative to HIV-positive among the women insisting on condom use – a very impressive result.

Why has this programme been so successful? We believe that making the women themselves responsible for the programme has been the main factor. This was reinforced by our methods; we took the services to the people and mobilized the community. The community responded with a high level of participation.

Making condoms easily available was the second important factor. This depended greatly on the support of the health education services.

Thirdly, we succeeded in reaching the clients indirectly through the women. The women thus proved to be powerful agents of change, and important motivators of the men.

It is gratifying that women who were already infected with HIV still insisted on the use of condoms. They had been educated to such a level that they appreciated the need to protect the client.

This study provides convincing evidence that targeted educational programmes on AIDS in Africa can bring about important changes in sexual behaviour. This reduces the risk of transmission of the AIDS virus. However, such programmes cannot be successful unless they are an integral part of a country's total health care system, particularly its primary health care component.

This work is part of a large study being carried out in collaboration with the following: F. A. Plummer, J. N. Simonsen, D. W. Cameron, and A. R. Ronald, Department of Medical Microbiology and Medicine, University of Manitoba, Canada; M. Bosire, Centre for Microbiology Research, Medical Research Institute, Nairobi, Kenya; S. Wanjiku and J. O. Ndinya-Achola, Department of Medical Microbiology, University of Nairobi, Kenya.

The Hot Rubber Story

ROGER STAUB

Mr Roger Staub of Switzerland, formerly a schoolteacher and now a consultant with the Federal Office of Public Health in its AIDS prevention and control programme, describes a dynamic campaign to persuade male homosexuals to adopt sexual practices that prevent transmission of HIV.

Three years ago in Switzerland, AIDS and rumours about AIDS began to cause great alarm, above all in the homosexual community. Some groups of this community wanted to take swift preventive measures. They decided to talk to other homosexuals about condoms, for it was already known that the virus is transmitted by intercourse. While some still remembered their youth and the protests of the girls when they were shown a harmless bit of rubber, most of them had never used condoms, not having any fears about pregnancy.

Fast action was needed, and the first thing they did was to distribute a simple booklet on safer sex, pointing out the dangers of penetration without protection. To help gays make their choice in what was to them a new area, this advice was accompanied by an advertisement for a well-known brand of condom. The meeting between these two worlds was effected through exchange; the manufacturer paid for the advertisement, not in cash but in samples, thus enabling 5000 samples to be distributed with the booklet.

Still, gays were not very keen on the idea of using condoms; they felt a sort of repugnance for this object, which they thought had been consigned permanently to oblivion. But even though this first experiment was not a great success, it did show the way ahead: the organizers must not try to exploit fear or ask people to give up an established practice. The change called for must appear simply as an adaptation, so that it would be widely accepted. It was thus decided to direct efforts towards a publicity campaign aimed at making the condom familiar and even smart and fashionable. Gays in the advertising profession joined forces with the initial group to help carry out this campaign. The volunteer professionals recommended that the information work should be supplemented by a marketing campaign based on solid realities. That meant having the best product, the best design, and as many easily

69

accessible sales outlets as possible. As a back-up to all this there had to be continuous publicity designed to reach all segments of the homosexual population.

Finding the right product required no more than a little common sense. What prostitutes used with success could be readily adapted. The product existed, but was of a rather clinical whiteness. A number of tests had to be conducted to develop a logo. The first one tried failed to get the entire target population to identify with it. The second achieved very wide acceptance; it was attractive without carrying too many connotations. An English name was chosen to cope with the problem of Swiss multilingualism and appeal to the cosmopolitan feelings of gays; product and logo were united and from the union came a trademark and also a distributing firm, the Hot Rubber Company. In November 1985 the Hot Rubber Company began selling Hot Rubbers in their definitive form at the price of one Swiss franc for two. The entire profits of the company were reinvested in the prevention campaign. The results were not slow to appear. Although those who tested the product during its development had not been impressed, when they tried it in its final version they found it finer and safer and the level of sensation high. In a word, they were won over; the Hot Rubber was made for them.

The product was there; it had to be brought to people. Bars and saunas, meeting-points for gays, were obvious distribution points. The first stage was to convince managers and owners to agree to the sale of Hot Rubbers in their establishments. After more than two years of effort it has now become possible in certain bars to order "a beer with" and be served beer with two condoms; some saunas make them available free of charge. Constant efforts are exerted on the publicity front. Every month a new poster comes out, intended for bars and saunas. The aesthetic presentation is different each time, making a more personalized identification possible. These regular renewals also provide a topic of conversation among the gays.

As a back-up to the publicity, and since the product is a new one, an instruction sheet on the use of the Hot Rubber has been issued. It tells the history of the condom and explains its use without prudery. Several sentences from this instruction sheet were re-utilized by a chain-store when it launched its own product.

In addition to observing the reactions of the people concerned, we undertook some spot evaluations. A survey conducted among gay circles in Berne after one year of campaigning showed that to the question, "What is the Hot Rubber?", 90% of those polled answered: "a condom" or "the gay condom".

The trend of sales figures also speaks for itself. The product came on the market in November 1985; in 1986, 125 000 condoms were sold. In 1987 sales stabilized at around 300 000; this figure should be seen in the context of the 6800000 inhabitants of Switzerland, some 100000 of whom may be regarded as potential customers. This levelling-off of sales may be accounted for by the fact that in the same year the national AIDS information and prevention campaign was getting under way. Major supermarket chains then began to offer products comparable in price and quality to the Hot Rubber. Anonymous purchase of condoms, as of milk or chocolate, became possible.

A national survey conducted in the summer of 1987 to determine what changes had taken place in the behaviour of homosexuals since the advent of AIDS showed that 85% of the persons polled had changed their sexual behaviour. The main changes were fewer partners, with a tendency towards monogamous union, and adoption of the basic rules of safer sex: anal intercourse with protection, and no sperm in the mouth.

Among homosexuals 75% say that they buy condoms. The Hot Rubber Company, bars and saunas, large stores and department shops are their main suppliers.

The efforts of the initiators of the campaign of prevention and publicity have not been in vain, the great majority of reactions having been positive from the start. Systematic evaluation has amply confirmed the results inferred from individual testimony. It is striking to find that in three years 75% of a well-defined group have changed their behaviour, especially since condoms were hardly ever used by the group.

The fact that the existing structures of an established community – specifically, bars and saunas – were utilized has certainly been conducive to individual acceptance of responsibility. Thus, instead of being induced by panic into deserting such places, the gay community have been given an opportunity to change their behaviour. Last, but not least, it was self-proclaimed gays who took responsibility for informing their community, and this certainly contributed to the fact that the instructions on safer sex were accepted as preventive and not repressive.

Clearly the campaign has to continue, with the object of raising within a very limited time the percentage of condom users among Switzerland's gay community to 100%.

It should, however, be stressed that the Hot Rubber campaign is only part of preventive work among the homosexual population of Switzerland, and only one of the Swiss programmes being conducted under the slogan STOP AIDS.

Overview of Part III Presentations

JAKE OBETSEBE-LAMPTEY

My task now is to draw lessons from the enormous range of strategies, messages and materials we have seen this morning. Before presuming too much, however, I thought I should quickly review the health promotion process and how each of our speakers fits into it.

Peggy showed how programme planning in New York City was based upon a detailed understanding of women in their different social roles – adolescent, sexually active adult, parent and sexual partner. A programme for "women" was not enough – individual materials addressed to each role-type were more effective than trying to reach all women as a single group.

Lone showed how Denmark used a careful study of adolescents and their life-style to plan a programme uniquely suited to them – vocabulary, music and speakers were selected solely because of their unique appeal to adolescents.

Grace took a step further into the implementation of a programme – the "how" of effective materials creation – showing that for her community the best materials emerged from exhaustive consultation, a traditional practice in aboriginal society, working with people to create relevant symbols, language and meaning.

Hans showed us how to reach a hard-to-reach audience, when he took us to Amsterdam where a "methadone bus" became the symbol for a well organized programme of support and resocialization of drug addicts.

Elizabeth showed how programme implementation can be carried out for another hard-to-reach group, female prostitutes in Nairobi. Again the real secret emerged from Elizabeth's experience: work with those affected – not for them; do things with people, not to them. And finally Roger showed how monitoring and evaluation make a good programme even better. Monitoring of attitudes of gay and bisexual men towards condoms in Switzerland showed that a special condom, the Hot Rubber, had to be developed.

I would repeat what I said in my introduction this morning: what we want you to take away from today's presentation is not an idea for a poster or a TV advertisement, but a process, for effective health promotion. This process begins with planning, finding out about your people and their high-risk behaviour, so that you can select specific target audiences. Then find out what your defined target audience already knows about AIDS, their attitudes towards AIDS, towards health, towards risks; their practices. Effective communication insists that we answer these questions with them; we must not assume that we know the answers already.

We must then involve the target audience in creating messages that will lead to change. There is a difference between knowledge and action – to tell someone that AIDS KILLS probably will not affect his behaviour. To communicate with the person and his or her peers in language and images that they understand can give them the opportunities and mutual support that may lead to change.

To admit that we do not always understand our fellow countrymen is not disgrace. After all, many of us with teenagers realize we do not always understand our own children. Yet we nurtured them, they are of our blood, they live with us. Others are not so close, so let us avoid the pitfall of assuming that because we are of the culture, of the country, we have the answers already.

A message, however good, that is not seen or heard cannot, by definition, be effective communication. The cultural sensitivity of sexual transmission and the taboo nature of some high-risk behaviours inhibit our ability as communicators to deal with the specifics of prevention: how, when, and with whom. These are difficulties that will be overcome with planning, creativity and the involvement of members of the target audience to be reached. In delivering messages it also helps to avoid clutter, to concentrate on one message at a time and benefit from repetition.

Effective health promotion guides itself with monitoring and evaluation. The planning process should set measurable objectives. Formal and informal, structured and unstructured, monitoring of progress in reaching these objectives will provide the direction for growth and change. Evaluation will reveal what we got right and what we got wrong. Mistakes will be made, but mistakes are only bad if they are left unrecognized and uncorrected.

Finally, I would repeat what you all know – AIDS affects us all; it is a challenge to every one of us in this room to provide the leadership and the resources necessary to help people all over the world protect themselves from HIV infection.

PART IV

The Critical Role of Counselling

Counselling is a means of mobilizing the psychological, social, and material resources of people with HIV infection or AIDS and of their close associates, as well as of the health workers and others concerned with their care and support. It offers psychological and social support, assists in modifying risk behaviour, and seeks to maintain HIV-infected persons as functioning members of their families and society. It aims at minimizing psychosocial and physical disability, and preventing further transmission, thus complementing and reducing the need for medical care.

Dr Manuel Carballo, Chief, Social and Behavioural Research, Global Programme on AIDS, WHO, presents the rationale of counselling in AIDS control and prevention, the principal needs it meets, and what it involves in terms of organization and education.

Introduction

MANUEL CARBALLO*

AIDS presents a new and unique type of challenge to health and social welfare services. Few diseases have involved, on such a broad geographical front, such a combination of physical and psychological stress as that associated in all societies with HIV infection and AIDS. No disease has highlighted, to the extent that AIDS has done, the close symbiosis between the individual and the community and the need for each to protect and support the other.

In the seven years that have elapsed since AIDS was first recognized it has become clear that those who are infected or have developed HIV-related diseases experience an extraordinary range of biological, psychological, and social problems. However, it has also become evident that AIDS can be prevented through informed and responsible behaviour.

While the long-term task will be to determine what mix of medical interventions is most appropriate and effective in protecting against infection and in the treatment of disease, the immediate challenge is concerned with how HIV infection can be prevented and, where necessary, managed, at the individual, family, and community level. It is also concerned with the type of positive social environment in which management of the disease can be made most effective.

Counselling, we believe, is one of the key components in any strategy to prevent HIV infection and provide care for HIV-infected people, including those who have AIDS. It is an interpersonal interaction and dialogue between a client and someone who is trained and skilled in counselling and at the same time well-informed about HIV infection and AIDS. While the value and importance of counselling is felt at the social level, its most important contribution is at the level of the individual and the family.

Individuals who learn that they are HIV-infected must be able to turn to some source of professional advice. Who is in a position and will help them to handle the initial fear and panic that so many people feel when

* Chief, Social and Behavioural Research, Global Programme on AIDS, World Health Organization, Geneva.

they discover they are infected? Where will they get the type of support needed to ensure that the changes in their life that will be needed can be carried through? If and when their resolve weakens, when they suffer rejection or humiliation or are discriminated against, where will they get personal support, continuing guidance, and help? When they need health and social services, who will help them discover what is available and ensure that they have access to them? Who, when others abandon them out of fear and ignorance, will still be able and willing to provide the time and support required? In almost all countries, counselling and the counsellor will have to be the source of the continuing technical and psychosocial support that will help in behaviour change, prevention of HIV transmission, and adaptation of the persons affected to the circumstances.

Many caring professions have in one way or another developed and used counselling skills and techniques. Counselling is certainly not a new kind of service. In the HIV epidemic, however, a new application of the principles and practice of counselling is called for in all routine social welfare and health activities. Counselling in the context of the HIV epidemic, moreover, stresses ideological commitment to the continued integration of HIV-infected persons within the wider community in a way that is economically, intellectually, and socially meaningful. At the same time it seeks to maximize the contribution that all individuals can make to the control and prevention of HIV infection through informed and responsible behaviour.

Counselling is essentially a response to four principal needs. The first is the need to provide psychological and social support to infected persons. Today this has become all the more difficult because stress and fear are almost synonymous with HIV infection and AIDS. AIDS primarily affects an age group which has traditionally been the least vulnerable to disease and death. As a result, anger at having been infected and fear of loneliness, of being stigmatized and rejected, and of becoming isolated are not uncommon. Feelings of loss of control, loss of autonomy, self-blame, and guilt contribute to anxiety and depression, further weakening people's ability to look after themselves and their families. The role of counselling is to strengthen the individual's control over everyday situations, the individual's responsibility to society, and society's responsibility to the individual. For, as infection progresses, the balance of responsibility will tilt from that of the individual to society for the prevention of HIV transmission, to that of society for the care of the individual who becomes too ill to function alone.

The second major need is to impress upon individuals and groups that changes in behaviour are required, indicating those that are acceptable, realistic, and feasible. Counselling closely complements other education and information measures aimed at preventing the spread of HIV. When education and information are directed at specific groups and presented in ways that respect their demographic, cultural, social, and psychological characteristics, they can be successfully used to explain and justify the need for behaviour change and risk reduction.

To be effective, however, information and education must first of all be accepted and then acted upon. Individuals vary in their capacity to deal with new information according to their personal background and the social pressures to which they are subjected. Many of the people and groups expected to make changes in their behaviour on the basis of the information and advice they receive will require active day-to-day support and encouragement that takes into account their background characteristics as well as the particular behaviour in question.

The third need to which counselling responds is to ensure the continued economic, intellectual, and social productivity and integration of HIV-infected persons within the larger framework of family and community. The belief that those who are infected are unemployable, should not be given educational opportunities, or should not be allowed to remain socially active would be as great a threat to society as a whole as it is to the individual or group concerned; families, friends, and acquaintances would suffer unnecessarily and society would be burdened with avoidable economic and welfare liabilities. HIV infection for the most part strikes an age group at the height of its economic, intellectual, and social productivity. The loss to society from actions based on such beliefs and the additional stress of rejection of the individual or group would be both irrational and counterproductive. One of the purposes of counselling, therefore, is to reinforce the continued and productive integration of HIV-infected persons by supporting the individual and those around him and by mobilizing appropriate realistic responses from the community. In this regard, the counselling of infected persons is linked to a much broader social purpose.

Fourthly, counselling responds to the need to minimize psychosocial and physical morbidity while reducing the burden on medical services when the type of care needed may not be medical in nature. Timely and effective counselling helps in the management of many of the psychological and physical health problems of HIV-infected persons, and thus can limit the need for clinical care.

There are several indications for counselling: when individuals are considering or being recommended for HIV-antibody testing; after testing when individuals receive the results; when apparently healthy individuals are found to be HIV-infected; after a diagnosis of AIDS or an AIDS-related condition; and when testing is not possible but an individual is believed to be at high risk of HIV infection. For each of these the individual's needs and those of his associates are likely to be different, and the counsellor's task will vary accordingly.

One of the principles of counselling is that a rapport must be carefully developed between an individual and a trained counsellor in a way that encourages problem-solving, the taking of responsibility for new behaviour, and adaptation to the notion of infection and illness. It is a relationship that requires trust, empathy, and time. It involves mobilization of necessary support from the health and social welfare system. In the context of AIDS, in which the progression from infection to disease can be long, counselling must maintain this relationship and ensure continuing support; interaction and support can mean the difference between successful and unsuccessful control and prevention programmes.

Counselling has for long been part of the management of other diseases, both chronic and acute. However, applying it systematically to the prevention and control of a disease is new. In a dramatically new manner, related directly to the epidemiological and social aspects of AIDS and HIV infection, counselling has become a critical part of the global AIDS strategy and of national AIDS prevention programmes. It is already teaching new lessons about the prevention and management of disease, lessons that will be directly applicable to other health conditions.

In every society there are already people who have been trained in counselling or who have acquired counselling skills. When possible, these people must be asked to participate in HIV counselling to help, together with those who are at risk, to organize new training programmes and develop plans to provide counselling services.

Where there are still too few trained counsellors, new training programmes will be needed. Fortunately in most communities there are people who, without formal training in counselling, possess many of the characteristics and skills required. These people must now be called upon and given clear accurate information and guidance about HIV infection and AIDS so that they can participate more fully in the counselling process.

What organizational forms counselling will take depends on HIV epidemiology. Where HIV infection is rare, counselling will be oriented to the prevention of high-risk behaviour. With a high prevalence of HIV infection, counselling must be concerned with both prevention and support. In any case, HIV-related counselling must always be an integral part of the broader health and social system.

In summary, we believe that counselling is the key to an innovative and powerful AIDS prevention and control strategy. In addition to bringing new techniques and knowledge to bear upon the control and prevention of AIDS, it may also have future application to many other health problems. To support countries in taking up this challenge, the Global Programme on AIDS is preparing a series of guidelines and training materials and organizing training workshops. Technical support is also available for the planning and development of national counselling programmes and strategies. We look forward to responding, together with countries, to this challenge and opportunity and assessing how counselling can be systematically and most effectively incorporated into national programmes.

Counselling Before HIV Testing

BENJAMIN HARRIS

Dr Benjamin Harris is Chief, Psychiatric Department, John F. Kennedy Medical Center, Monrovia, Liberia. He focuses here on the counselling of individuals who are considering taking a test for HIV antibodies. Irrespective of the question of a test, counselling is essentially geared to promoting non-risk behaviour.

HIV infection and AIDS are everyone's problem. No one is immune. Although the risks may vary, it is probably true to say that everyone is exposed to some degree of risk, some more so than others. Ever since the recognition of AIDS, of its principal modes of transmission, and of its serious social and health consequences, WHO has proposed counselling as a key strategy in its control and prevention. This includes attenuation of psychological and social morbidity.

Counselling plays an important role throughout the progress of HIV infection. Here I shall deal primarily with aspects of counselling that are particularly relevant to the pre-test period, when an individual who has not yet been tested for HIV antibodies is considering taking such a test. It is a period in which the role of counselling is to explore and settle a number of issues relating to why the individual is seeking to be tested, the nature and extent of his previous and present risk behaviour, the psychosocial implications of the test for him, and the steps that need to be taken to prevent him from becoming infected or from transmitting infection.

A variety of factors may contribute to seeking a test. In some cases individuals may be asked to be tested as part of employment or insurance regulations. In others they may simply be interested in knowing what their health condition is in general and, as part of this, their serostatus with regard to HIV infection. Unfortunately, the information that has been available to many people on the subject of AIDS has created irrational fears and concern. Many of those who come forward for testing do so in a context of agitation and anxiety. Psychiatric disturbances are not unusual during this period, in association with a morbid fear of HIV infection.

In some countries considerable numbers of people have come forward to be tested for HIV antibodies with no previous medical history or indication of previous high-risk behaviour. Often referred to as the "worried well", they place an immense burden on testing facilities and staff.

Depending on the society, a variety of cultural pressures and values may make test-seeking difficult or easy. Political and legal considerations may also play an important role in determining whether a person seeks to be tested and whether there is excessive anxiety associated with his action.

In some areas testing may not even be available, even though the area may be one of high AIDS prevalence, and the initial contact may represent the first the individual has with the health care system.

Counselling is fundamental before a test

Before testing, the importance of counselling is that it permits comprehensive assessment of the individual's risk background, psychological condition, and ability to deal with the results of the test and needs in the post-test period. In a way, counselling is the first level of screening. It requires discussion of the known modes of transmission and the particular behaviour that is likely to put the individual at risk. In assessing the risk, the counsellor considers the client's sociocultural context and is sensitive to, and aware of, cultural issues and culturally related risk factors.

There is no cure for AIDS. The possibility of developing a safe and effective vaccine to control the spread of the virus is still a long way off. The most important and effective strategy for controlling the spread of infection at present is through counselling bringing about positive behaviour changes that emphasize safer sex and awareness of high-risk behaviour. The primary reason for exploring risk issues in the counselling process is therefore to assist individuals to become conscious of how behaviour is related to health and disease and to learn how to modify this relationship.

Change in behaviour (especially as it relates to high-risk sexual practices) may appear to be simple. However, it is by no means easy. Well-established lifestyles and practices can be extremely difficult to change, especially if concepts of masculinity or femininity are closely associated in the local culture with sexual activity. Similarly, among individuals using drugs intravenously, or, indeed, where there is any drug abuse that involves collective and group support, a change in behaviour is all the more difficult because of the peer group pressure that is inevitably brought to bear on the individual.

Pre-test counselling attempts to clarify problems, settle issues, and eliminate misunderstanding by providing factual information. One of its first tasks is to make sure that the client is told as clearly as possible what the difference is between being seropositive and having AIDS.

All too often the stress experienced by the public, and certainly by those who are seropositive, is related to the confusion between HIV infection and AIDS; they assume that infection necessarily means the rapid onset of fatal illness, when clearly it does not. It is vital to emphasize, for example, that the test does not diagnose AIDS but detects antibodies to the AIDS virus. Additional information needs to be given on test specificity and sensitivity. Experience with AIDS-related counselling has shown that at some point most people want to know their chances of developing the disease if they take the test and if it is positive. Information on the natural progression of the infection needs to be provided sensitively and in a way that is easily understood. There also has to be an explanation of the latency period between the time of infection and the appearance of antibodies and consequently of the fact that a negative test result does not mean that the person tested is necessarily free from infection.

The development of responsible and effective coping skills is an important objective of pre-test counselling. We sometimes explore with the client the possible personal reactions to being positive or negative and the serious psychosocial ramifications of a positive test result. At some point role-playing exercises can be effectively employed in helping to look at this issue together with the client. Seropositivity can adversely affect employment, the taking out of insurance and, ultimately, status in the community. Confidentiality of test results is consequently vital, and the pre-test counselling phase must emphasize that this confidentiality is implicit in the relationship with the counsellor and will be respected at all times.

Pre-test counselling is also directed at the possible disadvantages of a negative test result. The false sense of security caused by a negative test result in an exposed individual who has not seroconverted always needs to be taken into consideration. A true negative result may equally present problems. This is exemplified by a 21-year old male, at high risk, who was so relieved by a first negative result that he went on an indiscriminate sexual spree. A further negative result six months later was followed again by sexual activities with a total disregard for safe sex practices. At a subsequent re-test about six months later he was found to be seropositive and has since been diagnosed as having AIDS.

Pre-test counselling also involves assessing how best to prepare the immediate circle of family and friends, who will inevitably be affected and who could be called upon to help. If the initial assessment suggests that the individual is at high risk, it is sometimes useful to help prepare them for involvement in the support network by informing them of the plan to take the test and the chances of its being positive. Community resources, which may include voluntary groups and self-help organizations, need to be identified. Determining whom to tell is not always easy and must always be done by the individual himself or herself.

Indeed, deciding to tell anyone has to be the individual's responsibility, and only his or hers. Pre-test counselling is the best opportunity for raising this issue, but only as a possibility and with an offer of support in arriving at a decision. The counsellor needs to bear in mind that it is those who are sometimes considered closest to the individual who may react the most negatively. Care therefore needs to be taken in this initial period to have a clear picture of what the response might be and what the real relationship is between the individual concerned and his or her most intimate associates.

It must always be borne in mind that counselling is geared to achieving a change in behaviour, irrespective of any decision about taking the test, of the outcome of the test, or even of whether testing is being considered. Moreover, the ultimate decision about whether to take the test is not the counsellor's to make. The decision should always rest with the client. The counsellor's role is to assist the client in exploring the issues, solving his or her problems, making the decisions that best suit his or her particular needs, and deciding whether the test would help in making other decisions.

There has been considerable discussion about the pros and cons of compulsory testing. Perhaps a more worthwhile and productive discussion would concern the pros and cons of compulsory counselling, since it is this that will ultimately bring about constructive change and lead to successful prevention and control of AIDS.

Counselling After HIV Testing

GLORIA ORNELAS HALL

Dr Gloria Ornelas Hall, Secretariat of Health, Mexico, is Director of the National Information Centre on AIDS, Mexico City. She draws on the extensive experience of the Centre with post-test counselling of HIV-infected persons and their sexual partners and families.

Much has been done to combat AIDS. But, in spite of the success of the many national and international intervention strategies and endeavours, the number of cases continues to rise at an alarming rate. It has not been enough to provide information; education is needed. Patterns of behaviour must change and support must be given to sustain the continuity of the change.

Mass information campaigns have on occasion saturated the media, at the expense of credibility. People no longer readily accept media messages of prevention. We need to reinforce existing measures on a new front, by offering individuals a face-to-face opportunity to assess their personal situation and by adapting counselling to their needs. That is our day-to-day experience at the National Information Centre on AIDS that has been established by the health sector in Mexico. We provide information on a permanent telephone call line and offer screening tests and counselling anonymously and totally free of charge. Those counselled include not only the population groups most at risk, such as homosexuals, bisexuals, prostitutes, drug addicts, and their families and partners, but also students, teachers, doctors, and people such as you and me, for unfortunately there is no group that is not affected by AIDS.

Our experience in post-test counselling in Mexico is an example of the type of approach that can be taken at a national level, and of how the principles of counselling can be observed even though unusual and unconventional methods are used. We view counselling as caring, caring enough to listen, to understand, to help deal with HIV infection and AIDS. It is a question not just of responding with good intentions but of offering up-to-date professional skills so that seropositive individuals can be assisted in problem-solving, in changing their behaviour, and in learning to live meaningfully with HIV infection.

Our centre is located in an old colonial house away from any institutional or official buildings, where people can feel free to come for help without fear of scrutiny by the authorities.

The experience of our programme was that at first people would just come in for information. Then it was risk groups that were being referred for testing. Later we were counselling HIV-infected individuals. Increasingly it was the symptomatic AIDS patient we were seeing; and it was not long before we were being asked for funeral guidance. Now we are counselling some of the sexual partners of those infected, whom we had previously seen in the waiting-room and who are now themselves infected. So we experience the day-to-day growing magnitude of the HIV epidemic and share its effects with those who owing to it are so often shunned by society.

AIDS is a deadly sexually transmitted disease and therefore gives rise to social panic, stigma, and rejection. Thus, when people are faced with the possibility of being HIV-infected they have a tendency to flee reality through myths and evasive fantasies. It is at this point in the HIV infection process that the value of post-test counselling becomes most evident. We have found that coping differs totally according to social, cultural, and economic background. HIV infection and AIDS may affect homosexuals, prostitutes, or drug addicts, low-income, middle-income to high-income individuals, or other than minority groups. Counselling programmes then have to respond to the various needs and characteristics of each person, adapting the message to his or her understanding.

We have, for example, discovered subcultures in minority groups where sexuality enhances self-destructive tendencies because of culturally determined feelings of guilt and shame. Many have been marginalized socially and their ignorance adds to their economic deprivation, leaving them with few resources to deal with the added burden of AIDS. Here post-test counselling must ensure that these individuals have immediate support and reassurance after a diagnosis of HIV infection; this may possibly prevent them from engaging in antisocial and personally disruptive behaviour. A counsellor must be able to detect their crippled defence mechanisms and help build them up to cope with HIV infection. If they have been discovered in the pre-test assessment, and empathy and good working relationships have been established with a counsellor, we recommend that the same counsellor should inform them of the test results.

We insist that counsellors be previously trained and that the training include role-playing exercises that place them in their client's shoes. We feel that not enough has been done to deal with medical and paramedical fears about AIDS or, indeed, about other communicable diseases. The front line against this deadly epidemic will be reinforced by the application of sound psychological techniques only when all counsellors have faced and resolved their own personal fears. What would *we* feel if we or our family were HIV-infected? Only then will we be able to treat the infected as persons with feelings and a need for kindness.

Our counselling is done in offices where sheltered space, intimacy, trust, and confidentiality can be guaranteed. Intimacy, we believe, can enhance rapport and overcome some of the problems of social distance that are inevitable where individuals are separated by a formal desk or the classic white uniform. Here post-test counselling may extend for months or years. Yet, it has to help set day-to-day objectives and share with the clients their problems of rejection; their shame and guilt; the continuing fear of letting others know; their isolation; their wanting to love and be loved, not through unromantic isolated relationships and emotionally empty "one-night stands", but through longer commitments that provide a more fundamental emotional involvement permitting and supporting behaviour change. All of the options theoretically open to the individual must be carefully weighed, taking his or her specific background and economic situation into account, and the range of support networks that can be called on, medical, legal, psychological, or economic.

It is through counselling approaches that take such factors into account that individual problems can be evaluated and solutions worked out. It is not realistic to tell prostitutes they have HIV infection without first analysing with them viable alternative sources of income and lifestyles. A homosexual cannot be expected to change his freely chosen sexual preference, but he can and must be told how to practise safe sex. The seropositive couple cannot be expected to stop making love, but counselling must ensure that they understand the risk of infecting offspring and are informed of ways of preventing pregnancy. Equally, one seropositive partner must be told of the risks the other partner is exposed to and the risk of an infected pregnancy. Likewise, intravenous drug-users should ideally be treated and encouraged to give up drugs, but experience compels us also to teach them how to sterilize syringes and, perhaps, at a later date, join in syringe exchange programmes.

Thus, through carefully designed post-test counselling, individuals can confront social values and modify and adapt their behaviour for their own protection and the protection of others. The goal of post-test counselling is to emphasize social responsibility and provide support for a change in risk behaviour. At the same time, it must uphold willingness to live and deal with an infection that may otherwise be attended by fear, ostracism, and possibly rejection, which could seriously impair the functioning of society at large.

Sexual partners and families too must be counselled, as HIV infection and AIDS also gravely affect them. Counsellors must calm their fears with solid information and practical guidance and support them in a common endeavour to ensure risk-free behaviour. Families must also be supported in coping with the effects of rejection. They must be dissuaded from marginalizing an HIV-infected family member; rather they must be persuaded to respond with responsibility to the commitment created by an oncoming illness that may require long-term care.

Unfortunately, a great number of our clients have a history of unstable relationships within their families, in their jobs, or with their sexual partners, and they therefore are often solitary. For them we have integrated group dynamics; HIV-infected individuals meet periodically and share experiences under professional guidance that reinforce their ability to cope with the fear of future suffering or death. Along with others an HIV-infected individual can confront AIDS, while prevention can be emphasized and epidemiological follow-up made possible that respects the individual's desire to be kept anonymous.

We have found that some of our most committed volunteers have emerged from groups such as these that had received counselling. They are creating new outreach groups that will open the way to social mobilization and help in the prevention of AIDS. One example is a deaf-mute promoter who has uncovered a silent subculture that depends on itinerant prostitution; another is a female prostitute who has been quite successful in teaching and promoting the use of condoms among her clients.

To fight AIDS effectively we must dare to look it in the face. This is what we do each time we face an HIV-infected individual in counselling.

Counselling of Persons with AIDS

DAVID MILLER

Dr David Miller is Senior Psychologist, Middlesex Hospital Medical School, London.
The counselling of persons with AIDS is concerned first with the crisis of diagnosis and then with the process of adjustment to a life under constant threat. Counselling is now in a position to benefit substantially from a growing body of research on how people cope with AIDS.

I would like to begin by expressing my thanks to three groups of people: first, to the World Health Organization and the Government of the United Kingdom for their gracious invitation to speak; second, to my colleagues, whose shared experiences and insights are reflected in what is described here; and finally, to my patients, with my deepest respect. Their courage, patience and sheer generosity at times of acute personal vulnerability has enabled us to learn much in the past six years. Our efforts and understanding stand as a memorial to their concern for the future welfare of their fellow men and women.

Counselling people with AIDS requires an awareness of the unique features that make AIDS different from other chronic diseases:

1. Often our patients are marginalized members of society, subject to prejudice and oppression. They will have internalized many negative social attitudes towards them, which may re-emerge after a diagnosis of AIDS.

2. Social and political opinion exerts considerable force upon how AIDS patients are diagnosed and managed and how people behave towards them. In particular, misinformed fear of social contagion has led to an often hysterical focus on sexual activities and restrictions on sufferers, at the expense of appropriate general HIV education and management.

3. Because the spread of HIV depends primarily on sexual and drug-injecting behaviour in young people, we as health professionals advocate behaviour change as a means of control.

4. Because of the universal association of AIDS and death, we counsel in a context of fear and hopelessness, despite the advances made in the understanding and management of AIDS. For these and other reasons it is easy to appreciate that HIV infection and AIDS are perhaps social

rather than medical phenomena, and why so many patient problems are not medical but psychological.

Counselling the person with AIDS involves two broad levels of engagement. The first concerns the crisis of diagnosis, the second the long process of adjustment to a life under constant threat.

The crisis of diagnosis

In Western experience patients seem to respond to a diagnosis of AIDS in the ways patients respond to other life-threatening illnesses such as cancer. Of course, the unique extra burdens of HIV, such as the stigma associated with homosexuality, intravenous drug use, and prostitution, and misperceived social fear of infection, are reflected in the familiar reactions to the diagnosis, which include shock, despair, grief, acute high-level anxiety, depression and withdrawal, anger, guilt, avoidance, and denial.

Such reactions are to be expected in the context of a perceived death sentence, but they are destructive, they undermine confidence and motivation to engage in constructive individual action. It is not surprising, therefore (especially with growing patient awareness of the possibility of AIDS-related dementias), that some patients react with suicidal impulses, especially if they are socially and culturally isolated, follow-up support and counselling are not offered or available, or the diagnosis is imparted in an insensitive manner to patients not carefully prepared for the possibility of such news.

The common theme underlying all these reactions is uncertainty. Uncertainty is a constant visitor in the life of the person with AIDS. Our own roles as health professionals play an important part in this; we cannot reliably forecast the course and prognosis of HIV disease for each individual, the availability or individual impact of new drug therapies (or their side-effects), or the levels of social tolerance or acceptance the new patient may expect to encounter. In short, we cannot help the patients reliably to see into their future; we can only decipher fragments from a short history and experience laden with prophecies of doom. We have to comfort our patients with the news that in these most important respects *they* are teaching *us*.

The process of adjustment

The highly complex process of adjustment to infection is determined by many variables: the patients' pre-morbid personality and psychiatric history, their range of and familiarity with coping experiences and skills, their motivations, relationships, family and social network, occupational flexibility and financial status, reactions to stigma and disclosures both of lifestyle and of HIV infection, their self-esteem and sense of personal identity, and their acceptance, control, and mastery of self. Adjustment also depends on the severity of the illness.

For example, many people with AIDS have had previous problems with major depression, alcohol and drug dependence, and anxiety disorders. The potential for a relapse is considerable and seriously compromising in the recently diagnosed, An increasing number of reports suggest that the stress of diagnosis and adjustment to it may lead in some to functional (as distinct from organic) psychiatric symptoms, although this is comparatively rare. However, we sometimes see psychotic features, paranoia, personality disorders, delusional states, and affective disorders, together with more common but no less disruptive psychological disorders such as chronic anxiety, reactive depression, hypochondriasis, and obsessive states.

The diagnosis may lead to a renewed expression of psychological problems associated with pre-AIDS lifestyle trauma. How such multiple loadings affect the response of individuals to AIDS may be crucial to their continued health, both physical and psychological.

Although such initial reactions and adjustment disorders may be quite transitory for many patients, for others they may come to characterize their life with infection or disease. Clinical evidence shows that greater difficulties are experienced by people who are socially isolated or have little family or peer acceptance, who have reservations or frank guilt about their sexuality or lifestyle, or who have poor accommodation and suffer additional insecurity in relation to resources, finances, and employment.

Intensity of psychological distress is also influenced by the diagnosis. Those with the AIDS-related complex (ARC) experience more psychological disturbance than those with AIDS or asymptomatic infection, because they are more uncertain about the likelihood of developing end-stage (and probably fatal) illness. Perhaps this explains why some patients express relief upon hearing the diagnosis of AIDS – at last, after months or years of slow decline and worry about the future, they know where they stand.

We are now at the stage where clinical counselling interventions can become more informed by the progress in research into the ways people with AIDS cope best with their condition. For example, studies emphasize that we should be encouraging our patients to engage actively in problem-solving and information-seeking and to participate in decision-making (particularly regarding their treatment options). The most successful counselling is that which encourages patients to take charge of their new circumstances. These and other studies emphasize that such an approach should be established as soon as possible after the diagnosis.

Research from San Francisco shows that as health becomes increasingly worse with AIDS, patient perception of the support available can change. This, along with the cognitive effects already resulting from chronic fatigue, weakness, and perhaps pain can lead to greater psychological distress. Where there is more perceived social support there is less hopelessness and depression. Conversely, lack of social support leads to an increase in depressive symptoms. Patients report that emotional support is crucially important for them, particularly when it comes from lovers, friends, and families.

It is vital also to consider the role of "significant others" in the care of people with AIDS. Carers and loved ones are our main community helpers. Yet good counselling necessitates that they too be informed and educated and supported throughout the post-diagnostic period, for the following reasons:

1. Loved ones may unwittingly add to the pressures on patients who may feel guilty or see themselves as a burden or a bore and therefore attempt to conceal their own distress in order to protect the loved ones (especially children) from the emotional or practical unheavals that often accompany chronic illness. In so doing, the patients may suffer greater emotional, psychological, and even physical distress.
2. Significant others may have misplaced fears about the risks of HIV transmission, which can easily be overcome with appropriate counselling and discussion.
3. Significant others have to live with the distressing consequences of the disease and of investigations and treatment just as do patients, and they too suffer from anxiety and the effects of prejudice. Studies show consistently that significant others run a far higher risk of developing chronic psychological disturbances than the patients themselves do.
4. The pressures associated with HIV infection may lead to family estrangement or, where family ties are maintained, to a conspiracy of silence never to discuss the true diagnosis with outsiders. These pressures can easily destroy families who lack support and information and, most important, the opportunity simply to talk to trained counsellors.

It is equally important to consider the social milieu of patients. If patients have known friends or others with HIV infection or AIDS, their response to the diagnosis may already have been formed. If friends or lovers have died of AIDS, fears may be intensified and lead to a greater demand on counselling. Worry over the ability of significant others to cope with the illness may also complicate the process of adjustment, especially where a patient's sexuality or lifestyle has not previously been disclosed.

A patient's social milieu can also be crucially helpful in management options. For example, community-based peer group support networks can maintain and develop counselling initiatives for people with AIDS and their significant others in the community. Such an extended family of supporters and carers also provides health services with major cost savings. No country's health systems can manage the burden of AIDS without voluntary peer-group and community-based support. Where they have tried to do so the services have been inadequate.

Research has shown unequivocally that it is when peer-based community support is allied to health system care that patients adopt and maintain low-risk behaviour best. However, this effect is obtained only if agencies are given motivation and government endorsement (including sufficient financial support), appropriate and consistent training, and the opportunity to cooperate meaningfully with medical management. It should not need saying that among the biggest handicaps to such potentially life-saving initiatives are social (and therefore government) apathy, indifference, or oppression, attitudes of moral superiority, and professional arrogance and territoriality.

To summarize, people with AIDS are required to grapple with the twin demons of uncertainty and adjustment, often in the context of social suspicion and scapegoatism. These create a constant tension that informs all the stages of disease following on the initial diagnosis. In counselling the person with AIDS, psychological distress must be managed alongside education and information about the control of HIV infection. However, with the diagnosis of AIDS comes a shift in the balance of social and individual responsibility. For the seronegative and asymptomatic seropositive person, the emphasis in counselling is on personal responsibility for future conduct and infection control. But with the onset of life-threatening disease society has the responsibility of acknowledging and supporting the needs of the person so threatened, including the responsibility of ensuring that impending decline is not cruelly complicated by social marginalization or, perhaps worse, indifference to the pain and loneliness AIDS creates. We have a responsibility to ensure that persons with AIDS have access to the widest possible range of resources so that they have the best care and comfort possible. If such resources do not exist, it is our responsibility to create them.

We know that, with AIDS, avoidance, denial, scapegoating, and moralizing kill just as effectively as the disease itself. AIDS has seen whole communities decimated. At the same time, whole communities have put aside their differences and risen to the challenge of affirming our humanity in all its variety and needs. Is it not time to say we are proud to take the opportunity to do the same? In doing so, we offer ourselves the best, and only, opportunity to stop the further spread of HIV. The communities from which we come are surely the obvious and most necessary starting-points.

PART V

Arming Health Workers for the AIDS Challenge

AIDS is making new demands on the health services and on the competence of health workers and has changed educational priorities. It has, *inter alia*, highlighted the need for intersectoral action and community involvement. These in turn make new demands on planners and designers of educational programmes.

Health workers engaged in the care of AIDS patients and in the control of AIDS have a special need for support. This mainly takes the form of information and training, and personal, psychological, material and technical support. The support is needed because, by reason of its complex medical, social and ethical aspects, AIDS imposes on physicians, nurses, and other health workers forms of stress associated with a sense of professional and personal inadequacy and fear of becoming infected.

Dr Daniel Tarantola, Chief, National Programme Support, Global Programme on AIDS, WHO, introduces this topic with an overview of the information, training, and other forms of support that health services and their personnel need for their tasks in AIDS control and the care of AIDS patients.

Introduction

DANIEL TARANTOLA*

AIDS is confronting health personnel with a widening range of new problems relating to biology, therapy, and behaviour. But what is most striking is that it has, by itself, led to the resurgence of many older problems that were familiar or at least suspected, which did not seem to require specific solutions and yet today seem to threaten and overwhelm us. Not a week goes by without the repercussions of AIDS on physical and mental health, on individual behaviour, and on society reminding us of our lack of vision, our negligence and our errors of judgement. Each time the patient turns to his doctor, society turns to its elected representatives, and the elected representatives turn to their government ministries and health departments for an answer or at least a sign of reassurance. Health personnel, sometimes well briefed, sometimes forced to interpret facts themselves, sometimes completely unequipped, are in the front line for action, but also for criticism. All countries in the world are desperately eager for information, education, and support as they face a challenge that has become a fact of everyday life.

This thirst for knowledge arises out of a deep-seated desire to do more and do it better, or out of the anxious questions asked by the public, by their elected representatives, and by the media. For health personnel, doing more and better means (i) being able to obtain information more easily and quickly, (ii) undertaking training, and (iii) receiving the necessary material and psychological support.

Information

Three aspects of information need to be stressed. The first is *quality*. The media, all too often criticized for helping to spread inaccurate news, are constantly faced with the risk that the information they collect may be less than reliable. Information may come from someone working in the health services somewhere in the world, or from one of the

---

* Chief, National Programme Support, Global Programme on AIDS, World Health Organization, Geneva.

many research centres, and it is not easy to assess with any confidence the extent to which the source of information has a mastery of the subject. For health personnel, this implies the need for greater ability to select good-quality information and to deal with the media with competence and a sense of proportion when supplying them with information.

The second aspect is *relevance*. In recent years, indeed even in recent months, a large amount and wide variety of printed matter intended for health professionals has made its appearance. Periodic bulletins, specialist journals, bibliographies and articles published in professional journals contain an abundance of information, which is becoming increasingly comprehensive. But it is sometimes hard to grasp, because of both its content and its form (AIDS is generating its own jargon). The relevant information must therefore be carefully chosen, either actively, when the individual selects his own mode of access to information, or passively, when the choice is made by someone else. In all cases, the purpose of the information selected will be to equip the health workers concerned with the optimum knowledge for carrying out their duties more effectively and reliably, and to provide or reinforce the information intended for the public, for elected representatives, and for those in government.

The third important aspect of information is *speed*. Here the developing countries are at a disadvantage. Long-distance data transmission facilities, direct access to the best sources of information, personal participation in congresses and conferences, or simply everyday access to a wide range of media enable the health personnel of industrialized countries to keep themselves constantly up to date. Elsewhere such opportunities are often scanty: information produced in the country itself does not circulate properly, and it takes weeks or months for information from abroad to reach a health team in a rural area. Moreover, national currency restrictions or prohibitive prices sometimes prevent staff from subscribing to international journals, and often it is not until the local journals publish an item that the information finally reaches its destination. How frustrated and helpless the doctor and nurse must feel in their health post when they learn from radio or television of some new developments but know they may not be able to find out more for a very long time!

Training

Training is the second component in the preparation of health personnel. No national health service employee, private practitioner, or voluntary health agency can fail to be involved with AIDS in the course of normal professional activities. The volume of training required is therefore immense.

It is essential to focus the training of the different categories of health personnel on the specific tasks expected of them and on the particular problems they will have to deal with. Curricula for health personnel are already top-heavy with subjects of doubtful relevance to the social and professional setting, while students are required to know far more than they need in some subjects and far too little in others. In the health sector, the principle of knowing more in order to know better has been very liberally applied, and educators have often lost sight of the fact that it is not just a matter of knowing, but rather of performing tasks and solving very specific problems. The advent of AIDS has generated a great deal of knowledge and new techniques, and it is the health sector's duty to re-examine its approach to staff training so as to prevent curricula from becoming even more overloaded than they already are.

AIDS is a health problem that has come to the forefront of worldwide concern, and in the process health personnel have found themselves under the spotlight before an audience seeking information and guidance. Clearly AIDS is a social and behavioural problem as well as a medical one. However, the health services have played a predominant role in making the general public aware of the nature and extent of the AIDS problem, and in every country they are continuing to prepare the ground for intersectoral mobilization for prevention and control of the disease. This is a leadership role to which the health services are unaccustomed and for which in many cases they are poorly equipped.

In the last few months – and this is a phenomenon as interesting as it is recent – health ministries have become unusually assertive in combating the lack of resources, the undeserved label of being consumers rather than producers, and the low priority often given to health considerations within the national political context. The ministries have swiftly set up technical advisory committees on AIDS, expanded them to include representatives of other ministries, and managed to gain a much better hearing from the highest authorities. This has happened spontaneously, and in many cases the health services have been faced with a new and urgent challenge, that of taking charge of intersectoral activities very much in the public eye and maintaining close cooperation and collaboration with other sectors that are more powerful, better equipped, and generally wield more authority. In the training of health personnel for the critical levels of the health system (which may very roughly be described as government, province (or district), and community levels), there is an urgent need to provide the skills and resources the personnel need to carry out their leadership and coordination duties. The professional dignity of those now responsible for this task is at stake. So is the credibility of the health services, both public and private, as a whole.

A final aspect of staff training concerns the need to get the community actively involved in prevention and control activities. AIDS made its appearance just when primary health care was successfully making the transition from concept to practice. AIDS is daily climbing higher up the list of health priorities everywhere in the world and it is obvious that if its transmission is to be prevented it is where transmission takes place, i.e., in the community, that the main work must be done. Moreover, the worst affected countries, whether industrialized or developing, favour the idea of community support for AIDS patients, which may include home treatment with family back-up and financial, emotional, social and religious support. In some countries, the AIDS patient's return to the village will stimulate closer collaboration between health service personnel and traditional practitioners. By learning to carry out AIDS prevention and control in the heart of the community, health personnel also learn to speed up the implementation of primary health care.

Material, technical, and psychological support

Our aim should be to provide health personnel with the most favourable conditions for carrying out their tasks. Such support is primarily of a practical nature; intensive health education cannot be undertaken without the necessary structures, staff, and channels of communication. This is an expensive and difficult undertaking, and it is well known that health education units are among the health services least well provided with human, material and financial resources. In some national programmes today the budget for education about AIDS is ten times the previous budget for all health education activities. This shot in the arm for a hitherto underprivileged area of endeavour should have a great many favourable repercussions on health activities as a whole, provided that the sudden expansion is properly planned and, of course, that additional financial resources are allocated at the national or international level.

Necessary material and technical support also includes the facilities needed by health personnel to detect the virus in donated blood and to sterilize medical and surgical equipment properly, so that health care procedures do not lead to virus transmission. It also means providing the staff with the equipment and supplies they need for their own protection. National programmes in developing countries are having to cope with a dramatic increase in requests for supplies of gloves, reliable and unbreakable laboratory and sampling equipment, and protective clothing. Here again, extra financial resources will be needed. The management of stocks, of distribution, and of replacement equipment will sometimes create major problems, but there will be a substantial spin-off for the prevention of other virus diseases, especially hepatitis B.

A legal framework and internal health service regulations are required to provide staff with clear guidelines on their responsibilities and respect for individual rights in regard to screening for HIV, monitoring of virus carriers, and treatment of patients. This legal and administrative framework will also provide an essential back-up for those who have to carry out their prevention and health care activities in settings where the public is liable to show opposition or even react aggressively. For many years health legislation has received very inadequate attention. The advent of AIDS calls for a very special effort in this area.

Confronted as they are by a health problem about which knowledge is still scanty, by patients – often very young – whose chances of survival are slender, and by an excessive burden of consultations and hospital admissions, health workers are exposed day by day to severe psychological stress. It is clearly becoming more and more difficult to persuade staff to remain in departments that see many AIDS cases. Some such departments have granted their staff shorter working hours, others have introduced a system of staff rotation, and still others have initiated group dynamics sessions in which problems of the relations between health care staff, their patients, and their environment are discussed. All of these initiatives need to be followed up most attentively, for obviously the physical and psychological stress to which health personnel are subjected does not create favourable conditions enabling them to provide their patients with the support they need.

Other aspects of support

Public and private bodies have already made a spectacular contribution to the expansion of an information support system for use by health personnel. WHO for its part has published a periodic bulletin (Update on AIDS), disseminated epidemiological and technical data in the *Weekly epidemiological record*, and produced and distributed technical documents on various aspects of AIDS control – such as guidelines for planning national programmes and reports on criteria for screening, new retroviruses and international travel. Many other reports are being prepared. A bulletin will shortly begin to appear periodically as a collaborative effort of WHO and the Appropriate Health Resources and Technologies Action Group (AHRTAG), a voluntary organization based in London. The WHO Division of Public Information and Education for Health, strengthened by staff specially assigned to the programme on AIDS, has collected a large quantity of audiovisual material produced in different parts of the world, which can be used to produce material properly suited to local situations.

Great use has been made of radio and television to pass on information to the general public as well as to health personnel. The Global Programme is at present establishing a telematic system which will complement similar systems already developed in several countries for essentially local or national purposes. The WHO system will enable a worldwide user network to have access to an AIDS data bank. Users of the network will have to possess an ordinary microcomputer connected to a telephone line. Talks are in progress with the association International Physicians for the Prevention of Nuclear War with a view to the network gaining access to a satellite launched by the USSR and whose frequencies would be put free of charge at the disposal of the Programme.

Numerous training courses, workshops, and conferences on AIDS have been held during the last few years, particularly in 1987. These activities have been concerned with very varied aspects of AIDS control, ranging from serological diagnosis of the infection and its clinical and psychological management to information and education. WHO for its part has brought together over 150 specialists in briefing seminars for consultants employed by the Programme. Two seminars of this type have been held in Geneva and one in Australia; in 1988 others will be held in the African Region, the Region of the Americas, and the Eastern Mediterranean Region. The seminars have made it possible to brief the consultants needed to carry out over 300 missions in various parts of the world between February and December 1987. Guides for trainers are being prepared for various categories of health personnel and personnel in other sectors. One such guide, for nursing staff, is to be published shortly.

Although WHO recognizes the advantages of an international exchange of participants in training activities, the Programme is concentrating its efforts on individual countries. Indeed, once trainers have themselves been well trained, the specific social and cultural features of national AIDS control programmes and the need to train very large numbers of people make it essential for the training to take place in the environment to which the participants are accustomed. The Programme furnished large-scale support to countries in 1987, obligating to the support of national programmes almost US$ 15 million, or about two-thirds of its total budget. A large proportion of the funds was devoted to strengthening the structures, educational activities, and equipment of national programmes. In 1988 a sum of US$ 40 million will be committed for activities in countries, while an increasing proportion of their national budgets will be assigned to AIDS control by the countries themselves. This effort must be sustained. Information, training, and effective support must be commensurate with the size of the AIDS problem and will require world mobilization over a long period.

Knowledge and Fear among Health Workers: The San Francisco Experience

PAUL A. VOLBERDING

Dr Paul Volberding, Chief, Medical Oncology and AIDS Activities Division, San Francisco General Hospital, USA, saw the first cases of the newly recognized disease now called AIDS. He explains in this paper why health care systems may need to be changed to cope with the medical complexities of AIDS and its associated social and ethical problems, what stresses AIDS care imposes upon physicians, and what may be done to support them psychologically.

The physician caring for AIDS patients undertakes a degree of responsibility and faces an array of problems greater than that pertaining to almost any other patient group. Not only is AIDS care challenging in its medical complexity but also the stigma and the social and political problems associated with the disease are forcing caring physicians to consider aspects of medicine in its wider context, that many had previously preferred to ignore. For example, will health care providers be affected by the social fear and discrimination associated with homosexuality and intravenous drug use? Can we organize and maintain a comprehensive and socially sensitive system of care for AIDS patients while many in our society continue to think of AIDS as someone else's problem? Can AIDS health care providers find the personal support they will need if they are to continue to see their best efforts fail to prevent tens, and soon hundreds, of thousands of deaths from this dreadful scourge?

We have already heard about the vital need for more accurate and timely information for health care providers. I should like to consider two additional needs if the medical community is to cope with the still growing threat of AIDS. One is the need to reorganize systems of health care to meet the unique problems of AIDS; the other is the need to develop and implement strategies of psychological support for AIDS providers.

None of us can completely escape the biases of personal experience. My remarks will undoubtedly reflect the fact that I work primarily with

103

homosexual men with AIDS in a city, San Francisco, that has been more supportive of this work than any other city in the United States. My patients are typically well-informed about their illness and comply with their treatment, and they have been able to mobilize an array of community-based resources that reflect San Francisco's inclusion rather than exclusion of homosexuals in the political process. Despite this somewhat parochial experience, I hope that we may still find some value in this discussion. If AIDS care is difficult even when there are many resources, how much harder it must be in other situations!

Ideally, the system of health care should be designed to meet the needs of the patients. To force an illness into an unsuitable system is at best inefficient and at worst ineffective in meeting patients' needs. AIDS, because of its medical complexities and associated social and ethical problems, does not fit easily into medical care as it has evolved in the past several decades.

The central and most obvious difficulty in organizing AIDS care is the multidisciplinary nature of the care. In AIDS any organ system can be the target of life-threatening infections or malignancies, and often several are involved simultaneously. Thus either the AIDS physician must be a particularly gifted and educated generalist, or a team of physicians must be assembled ready to deal effectively and in coordinated fashion with that wide spectrum of disorders. In addition to strictly medical problems, AIDS patients have psychosocial difficulties which the health care team must confront. AIDS patients are frequently young, have few savings, and because of medical problems or discrimination may lose their job, their home, and all too often their family and friends. Obviously the physician's care is of little value to a patient who is unable to find a place to live in or food to eat. Therefore the physician must ensure that these social services are provided – an addition to the burden of AIDS care.

Still another burden on the health care worker is that of the ethical problems posed by AIDS. For example, when is limitation of care or withdrawal of support ethically admissible for a patient who is young, has no one who can speak for him, and because of AIDS-related dementia is unable to express his own wishes? How should the physician involved in AIDS care react when colleagues refuse to assist in care because of their own beliefs or fears? What resources should be used in the care of AIDS patients with an apparently dismal prognosis when they may be needed for non-AIDS patients with a better chance of recovery? What are the ethical aspects of compulsory testing for antibodies and of quarantine and what role should the physician play in this often rather political debate? I pose these ethical issues as questions quite deliberately because I do not think we know yet how to answer them. This does not mean, however, that they are not practical questions or that we can avoid them, for they face us daily. And yet we find physicians poorly trained in medical ethics. This again, adds to the burden of the AIDS health care provider.

I have raised the subject of the stress on the physician in AIDS care, but before addressing it directly I shall summarize some components of an optimal health care system for AIDS patients. First, the system must be multidisciplinary, probably combining skilled generalists trained in AIDS with specialists in, for example, oncology and infectious disease. Secondly, individuals able to assist patients with their social, economic, and psychological difficulties should be included, as should skilled and practical medical ethicists. Finally, the system should use the resources available in the patient's community so as to control the growing burden on the acute-care hospital. In my own city, where we have seen over 5000 cases of AIDS, we have found that AIDS-dedicated inpatient units and outpatient clinics, staffed in part by representatives of gay community organizations, assume many of these tasks.

What are the stresses on the physician caring for AIDS patients (irrespective of the system of care) and how can we reduce them so that they do not limit the involvement of physicians? Let me briefly mention some general reasons why physicians have chosen to limit their involvement with AIDS. First, they may be intimidated by the rapidly growing medical complexity of AIDS-associated illnesses and the many diagnostic and therapeutic approaches available. Secondly, they may be afraid of becoming infected with HIV in the course of their occupation. Thirdly, like many others in our society, they may fear the behaviour, both sexual and drug-related, that accounts for much of HIV transmission – a fear that contributes to the discrimination against AIDS patients. Finally, they may feel unable to cope with the severe psychological stress of caring for the young, dying, disfigured, isolated patient so typical in this epidemic. I would maintain that, with an aggressive programme of professional education, we can limit the impact of the sense of professional inadequacy and the fear of HIV infection. I believe that education alone will not control discrimination, and that there are other things we might do as well to help physicians handle the stress AIDS care imposes on them.

We have already referred to some of the sources of stress. The patients are young, deteriorate physically and often mentally with a grim inexorability, and almost inevitably die. Can you imagine how great a burden this is for the physician who still, undoubtedly naively, enters the medical profession to cure the sick? How frightening it is when the patients who are dying are like the physician himself in so many ways, wear the same clothes, listen to the same music, have attended the same schools, and in some cases share the same sexual preferences! Have many of us reconciled ourselves so well to our own mortality for this sight not to cause pain and fear? And what must it be like to have come to know tens, hundreds, and perhaps soon thousands of people with AIDS, who have fought against and finally died of the horrible virus we call so simply HIV?

In San Francisco we have diagnosed thousands of AIDS cases, so perhaps it should not be surprising that we are also experiencing stress in response. I cannot tell you that we have found a way of reducing the stress. We do not yet even know the full extent of the problem. Some of the current attempts at reducing stress may however be mentioned; they range from efforts to distribute AIDS care throughout the community to more effective management of our own programme, and group therapy for staff at all levels.

One of the basic ways is to spread the stress by distributing AIDS patients as widely as possible without compromising the quality of their care. This may involve disseminating lists of physicians interested in AIDS care and establishing AIDS care services in many rather than a few hospitals. Using the educational approaches recommended by Dr Tarantola, all physicians must be encouraged to become involved, and hospitals should be similarly encouraged. For example, under the leadership of Dr Donald Abrams, we have held monthly meetings with community physicians who care for AIDS patients and are now organizing clinical research with them as well as sharing the latest AIDS information. We also distribute a newsletter of practical AIDS information without charge to all physicians in our region.

Many of the stresses I have referred to are increased because of the rapid growth in AIDS-related organizations as we try to keep up with the growing epidemic. The resultant stress gives rise in staff members (physicians and others) to feelings of isolation from co-workers and uncertainty about their own values. We feel that careful attention to communication within the organizations is vital for the control of this sometimes crippling stress reaction. We try to share our goals with our staff and solicit group participation in decision-making.

Even when other sources of stress are controlled to the best of our ability, how can we cope with our patients' suffering and death? Here we are just beginning. One of the most exciting of our recent efforts has been our collaboration with a group called the Center for Attitudinal Healing. Two members of this centre have led a group of ten of us for the past six months. From them we have begun to learn principles that seem applicable to our personal lives, as well as to our AIDS care organizations and the care of our patients. We have learned that anger and discrimination are expressions of fear, that there is no conflict if we choose not to participate, and that underlying much of our stress is fear of our own mortality. Taught by these and other lessons, we hope to continue to take care of our patients and yet remain healthy in all respects ourselves. These results have lead to the enthusiastic launching of a second similar group, and others will be started as our needs and resources permit. Unfortunately, along with education, stress reduction groups for AIDS health care providers are seen as luxuries rather than as essential elements in the control of the epidemic. If I can convince you of but one point today it would be this: AIDS places severe and chronic stress on health care providers, and if they are to maintain their own health and continue to provide effective care they must be provided with the resources needed to reduce the stress.

I have tried today to offer several ideas for your consideration. The complexities of AIDS care force us to reconsider our health care systems, ask ourselves whether our systems are functioning well, and be prepared to revise them to enable us to deal with the medical, psychosocial, and ethical problems of AIDS. I have also reviewed some of the reasons why physicians have chosen not to become involved in AIDS care, and action that can be taken through intensified professional education and new regulations or standards of conduct within our profession. Finally, I have reviewed the enormous stress of AIDS care and suggested several possible approaches to its control. Let us hope that we shall find qualities in ourselves and in those around us that will permit us to improve our efforts without forgetting the humanity we all share.

Health Workers, the Community and AIDS

Ms Mafama Omba Ngandu is Director, Paediatrics Department, University Clinic, Kinshasa, Zaire. Her paper describes the effects on a hospital paediatric department of the sudden appearance and growing numbers of infants and young children with AIDS – the fear of the staff, the resentment of parents and families, and the gradual development of new relationships and new rules for the hospital and the community.

It was at a conference on AIDS in 1983 that my colleagues and myself, health workers at the hospitals in Kinshasa, heard about this new problem from the experts who had come from the United States of America. My colleagues and I returned home convinced that this new disease was something of a curiosity and did not concern us directly, although it did have a number of complex and intriguing aspects. A year later, in 1984, a succession of courses and workshops taught us more about this problem and put us on our guard.

My first patient was an infant of 11 months born to a 24-year-old single mother. Admitted in a state of emaciation, with pneumonia which had been treated for over a month without success, persistent diarrhoea that did not respond to medication, and stomatitis, the infant was given a number of AIDS tests, all of which were positive. The infant died a few days later. We did not dare tell the parents what its disease had been. We would not have known what to say or do to prevent them reacting with panic, so we said nothing. As other cases were admitted day after day to the hospital, we were given protective materials such as gloves, overalls, and disinfectants, and we stepped up precautionary measures. This sudden issue of protective materials may have helped trigger the reaction of fear that quickly gripped the health workers in my department. Fear of infection made us keep away from patients with diarrhoea and from people who coughed or merely had simple skin rashes. Caring for patients, who were usually put in isolation, became increasingly difficult. The staff asked the patients' families to see to their personal hygiene, or put considerable pressure on doctors to prescribe remedies to be administered orally rather than by injection. There were obviously two groups confronting each other: the health workers on one side, the patients and their families on the other, with AIDS in between.

Things have progressed a great deal since 1984. The two groups have come much closer together as information and training have succeeded in conquering ignorance and fear. The fear of infection has now been reduced, although it persists among health workers in rural areas who have not yet benefited from the education programmes set up by the Coordination Bureau for AIDS Control established in 1987. In the hospitals of Kinshasa and the large towns of Zaire, health workers have learned to improve their technical efficiency and to provide the psychological support expected by patients and their families. Tact, prudence and patience are essential in the establishment of such good relations.

The patients, whose numbers are growing daily, wish to spend as little time as possible in hospital. The overloading of services, staff shortages, and overcrowded wards make the patients and their families wish to return home rapidly.

There is often a lingering fear of the disease among those closest to the patient, which prompts them to refuse permission for the screening of children, who are my main concern. When the family has been persuaded that the test is necessary, and if the result is positive, the news often causes great distress. Husband and wife engage in mutual recrimination or accuse us of having infected their child during previous medical treatment. Some parents disappear, abandoning their child, while others decide to face up to this new trial together, surrounding the child with all the care and affection they can muster at the hospital or in the village, depending on where the community provides the best physical and moral environment for confronting the problem.

The extent of the epidemic is such that the hospitals, which were already overcrowded, cannot accommodate all AIDS sufferers for lengthy periods. It is now essential to prepare communities to accept and provide services for healthy HIV carriers and AIDS cases. Our communities are capable of performing a number of tasks if health workers give them the necessary support. First, they need to be made aware of the disease and its modes of transmission, and of what behaviour puts people at risk. They should learn also how it is not transmitted. Examples from everyday life can be used to illustrate the situations where contact with an infected person entails no risk.

Secondly, communities must be informed about the system of referral for screening and where to go for advice and treatment. Where condoms are one of the methods of preventing the disease, the community must know where to obtain them and how to use and dispose of them. This information is given to carefully selected groups in such a manner that neither its content nor its presentation conflicts with tradition.

The community can play an important role in ensuring that health workers use appropriate procedures. The public can, for example, check with health personnel that needles, syringes, and any medical instruments to be used have been properly sterilized. One indication that this is feasible is that there are patients in Kinshasa who buy a sterile syringe for their personal use before going to hospital for treatment.

The community can also help prevent diseases that cause anaemia, which all too often leads to the need for blood transfusion. Parasitic diseases, malnutrition, and diseases of the blood, such as sickle-cell anaemia, can be combated by sustained primary health care work.

Finally, since AIDS has a direct effect on the community, education programmes need to be set up so that the community, far from stigmatizing and ostracizing people with AIDS, accepts and supports them. In this respect traditional medicine can play a very important role. It gives the sufferers hope and comfort and helps the community accept them and their families. However, traditional medicine is not always cheap; some families may be ruined financially by protracted illness and treatment. Modern medicine can be associated with this treatment in places without health care facilities, as long as a member of the community is familiar with the salient features of certain opportunistic infections and can dispense a few carefully selected drugs. Oral candidiasis, for example, can easily be treated in the home, thus giving sufferers some comfort and allowing them to eat. The distribution, storage, and supply of essential drugs, even cheap ones, are often very complex and we, as health workers, still have much to learn about logistics.

Nurses and health workers also have an important role to play in the education of members of the community who can take a prominent part in community care. These include in the first place the administrative and traditional authorities, without whose support nothing can be done in our countries, and, secondly, professional groups such as teachers, who must not only teach children about AIDS but also be prepared for the appearance of the disease among their pupils or their families. Finally, there are the religious authorities, whose assistance should be sought both in prevention and in the provision of the support needed by sufferers and their families.

In conclusion, health workers confronted with AIDS in the hospital environment must now adopt a more dynamic approach to the disease, attacking the problem at its source, i.e., in the community. The tasks we have described can be carried out in our villages and towns by those around the patients, as long as they are given proper instruction and continuous support and as long as health workers are well prepared and have the means to set up a programme of action.

Ensuring Safe Injection Procedures

NILTON ARNT

Dr Nilton Arnt is intercountry epidemiologist with the Pan American Sanitary Bureau in Buenos Aires, Argentina.

Hippocrates particularly enjoined physicians never to do harm. Medical injections can transmit AIDS. Health administrators, physicians, and other health workers have it within their power to eliminate the AIDS transmission caused by medical injections.

I am sure that many have heard people say in informal conversation about AIDS that they might eventually become resigned to AIDS acquired through a chosen sexual practice but never to that from a blood transfusion or medical injection. Quite apart from any moral considerations of guilt or innocence, such a widespread attitude underscores the dramatic confirmation AIDS brings us, as health service managers, of the cogency of the Hippocratic principle not to do harm. In this perspective, I invite you to reflect for a few moments on the medical actions that are directly associated with the possibility of AIDS transmission.

We can easily imagine the suffering caused by a mistaken diagnosis as a result of a substandard laboratory service, or the personal and family tragedy caused by a positive finding communicated without preliminary psychological and social preparation. It is equally easy to see the potential for harm of a blood transfusion or treatment involving the use of blood products. But the prospect of danger is not so obvious when we consider such a commonplace medical procedure as injection, possibly because the risk of AIDS transmission is very low. We cannot, however, be complacent. Rather, we should take the view that it is unacceptable that even a single case of AIDS should be caused by an injection given in a health service. Nothing can justify a tragedy of that kind. Resolute determination to see that it does not happen will lead to the introduction of some very simple measures that will have an overwhelming impact on health, for they will close the door not only to one route of AIDS transmission but also to hepatitis, abscesses, and other infections, thus increasing public confidence in the health services.

I should like to highlight three of the measures that are possible:

1. *Reduction in the number of injections*

We are convinced of the absolute necessity of about 25% of the injections given in many countries to children in the first year of life to immunize them against tuberculosis, diphtheria, whooping cough, tetanus, and measles; they prevent a million deaths among children every year. A large proportion of the other injections they are given – about 75% – have no legitimate justification; they are given on the false assumption that medicaments administered by injection are more effective than those administered orally. The elimination of unnecessary injections, which would be feasible through health education of the public and of health workers, would automatically lead to a reduction in the risk of HIV infection by this route. We have all heard stories of doctors whose patients have left them because they have not prescribed injections. There again health education is required.

2. *Provision of adequate injection equipment*

Three types of equipment are in common use: re-usable syringes and needles, disposable syringes and needles, and jet injectors. Re-usable needles are made of stainless steel. Re-usable syringes are made of glass, nylon, or plastic. Re-usable steel needles with plastic adaptors and re-usable plastic syringes are gradually coming to be preferred. They are unbreakable and will withstand autoclaving 50–200 times. Disposable syringes and the nozzles of disposable needles are also made of plastic, but of a less resilient type than is used for re-usable syringes. They become distorted when they are boiled or autoclaved. Jet injectors are precision instruments designed for the high-speed administration of a large number of injections. The tip of the injector is placed against the skin and the vaccine is ejected in a fine jet at high speed and penetrates the skin. No other instrument is needed.

Today we have new types of cheap re-usable needles and syringes, which are also suitable for special mass vaccination campaigns. As they are supplied already sterilized, they can be put to immediate use. The additional cost of procuring sufficient quantities to ensure that there is a sterile needle and syringe for every injection given during a vaccination campaign is offset by the twofold advantage that the long-term cost is lower and that the routine health services then have injection equipment for further use. Sterilization involves additional costs in equipment, time, and energy. Even so, re-usable plastic syringes are less expensive than disposable syringes. WHO has done studies that show these differences in cost.

The industrialized countries have mostly adopted disposable syringes, which are used once and then destroyed. This saves them the high cost of staff time required for sterilization, and there are proper facilities for the disposal of materials. In many developing countries, however, disposable needles and syringes cannot be recommended. In practice they increase the risk of infection, for two reasons:

- when discarded by the health services but not destroyed they end up in less qualified hands, and sterilization may be less than satisfactory;
- proper sterilization shortens the life of most disposable materials, and hence health personnel often do not sterilize them adequately.

The quantity of disposable needles and syringes required is 50–200 times greater than the quantity of re-usable supplies, which increases transport and storage requirements. It must also be remembered that some re-usable syringes and needles and sterilization facilities must be kept in reserve in case there are breaks in the supply of disposable materials.

3. *Proper sterilization practices*

If a sterilized needle and sterilized syringe are used for every injection, the risk of transmission of the AIDS virus and other infectious agents is eliminated. To ensure this, peripheral health services must receive both equipment and supplies and have the necessary knowledge to ensure that sterilization is carried out properly. This requires adequate funding, the training of health personnel, and certain managerial skills.

Autoclaving at a temperature of 121°C for 20 minutes is sufficient to destroy all the micro-organisms that cause disease. The immersion of needles and syringes in boiling water for 20 minutes does not necessarily kill all micro-organisms but does destroy most bacteria and the AIDS and hepatitis viruses. This is an acceptable method of sterilization when there are no facilities for autoclaving. Autoclaving can be carried out with apparatus that has recently been developed from the domestic pressure cooker and is specially designed for immunization centres.

Health workers cannot use the proper techniques unless they are trained to do so. Educational technology for this type of training is easily available, but safe sterilization requires an extra effort and training alone is therefore not enough; it must be reinforced by incentives and supervision to ensure that the extra effort is made.

As well as reliable equipment and trained and motivated personnel, there must be available essential supplies such as fuel. Even so, all these inputs will be effective only if they are supported by a good administrative system.

All this costs money. However, failure to eliminate the risk of AIDS transmission by injection cannot be excused on the ground of cost. Studies have shown that the cost of safe sterilization adds only 2% to the total cost of immunizing a child.

I should like to mention the following important points for your final consideration:

- WHO and UNICEF play an influential part in product development and are coordinating independent evaluation trials. The results are published and distributed to countries to provide them with guidance for their own decisions. UNICEF also has stocks of many of the items to which I have referred.
- WHO and UNICEF are acting for countries in the procurement of supplies and equipment. It may be possible to establish a global procurement scheme, with funding mechanisms along the lines of the Pan American Health Organization revolving fund for the purchase of vaccines.
- The WHO Expanded Programme on Immunization is coordinating a vast scheme for the training of health personnel in immunization. It could be further expanded to include all types of injection.
- Basic information and news of technological advances are passed on to countries through the regular newsletters published by special programmes. At this meeting we are launching the circulation of guidelines for efficient sterilization and disinfection against the AIDS virus.

In summary, we can say that all the conditions are met that enable health services to eliminate AIDS transmission through medical injections. It is political will that will serve as the catalyst to transform this possibility into practice. The commitment remains that we should do no harm.

Closing Addresses

Tony Newton, Minister for Health
Department of Health and Social Security, United Kingdom

Dr Halfdan Mahler, Director-General
World Health Organization, Geneva, Switzerland

Tony Newton

MINISTER FOR HEALTH, DEPARTMENT OF HEALTH AND SOCIAL
SECURITY, UNITED KINGDOM

As the Summit draws to a close, I would like to make a few remarks. I am sure you will agree that the Summit has been an excellent example of international cooperation. First, it has brought together an unprecedented number of ministers of health, as well as representatives of many international nongovernmental organizations, to exchange views and share experience. Representatives of 149 states have attended this Summit, nearly all of whom are ministers. This has provided a unique occasion to hear authoritative speeches and reports of the latest position and the action being taken in a large number of countries. In the formal presentations we have heard of the successes in AIDS education. In the private discussions we have had a chance also to hear about the pitfalls and difficulties. In both respects we can learn from each other.

Second, there has been an unprecedented level of agreement – indeed a universal consensus – that the whole international community must work together in seeking to prevent the spread of HIV infection. The London Declaration we have agreed on today focuses on and gives impetus to national and international action in the vital areas of education and prevention, and I hope you will give a further impetus to these efforts.

I wish briefly to highlight some points from the Declaration that strike me as particularly significant. First, we have recognized the need for information and education programmes as a vital element in national programmes for action; this indeed is a central theme of the Summit. These programmes must of course be designed to meet the needs of particular countries and to address both the population as a whole and different groups within the population.

Second, we have recognized the need for international cooperation and coordination and the central role of WHO in achieving this. We have charged WHO with a number of important tasks that are set out in the Declaration. These tasks will not be easy. Together we must now ensure that we provide WHO with the support and resources needed to carry this work through. And individually we must see that our own countries take all the necessary steps.

Third, we have recognized the need to acknowledge the rights and dignity of people infected with HIV and with AIDS. We must avoid the situation where infected people are excluded from society, stigmatized and discriminated against. And we must ensure that people with AIDS receive care and support of the same standard as we would extend to people who are sick for any other reason.

Fourth, we have recognized the need for governments, and in particular health ministers, to exercise leadership in carrying through their countries' AIDS prevention programmes. The Summit, and the sense of purpose that has been shown by everyone here, gives real cause for believing that this leadership will be given.

This Summit has given us the opportunity to learn, to share experience and information, and to join together in making a far-reaching declaration of principle on action to curb the AIDS epidemic.

The consensus achieved here on what is needed both nationally and internationally and the commitment that has been demonstrated towards taking the necessary steps make me optimistic that together we can achieve our aim.

In opening our proceedings the Princess Royal asked us to make this Summit work. As our programme draws to a close, I think we can claim to have done just that. And now we must ensure that our work here in London is followed by action at home.

Halfdan Mahler

DIRECTOR-GENERAL, WORLD HEALTH ORGANIZATION

I believe the exchange of information and experience at such a high level during the past two days has inspired all of us to become much more optimistic than we were that we can and will defeat AIDS.

The Declaration of this Summit is excellent. However, the true test of this Declaration and of our intentions is action. Therefore, within four weeks from today, I will be contacting you regarding the further steps of implementation which we all seek. This Summit, marking an important step along our common path, will be followed up with great energy and commitment. We must therefore make sure that the exchange of information becomes a continuing process everywhere and receives high public visibility in order to induce as widespread optimism as possible. We must make use of this Summit as a launching pad for a sustained AIDS communication programme throughout the world. You have designated 1988 as a year of communication on AIDS and I intend to promote an annual World Day of Dialogue on AIDS, the first to be on 1 December 1988.

What is the basis for my optimism? Much of it has been inspired by what I have heard at this Summit. It is conditional optimism – conditional on what you do when you return home. The conditions will be fulfilled:

- if you ensure the political commitment of your governments as a whole to fighting AIDS
- if you motivate your heads of state to take a personal interest in the fight
- if you mobilize leaders in all walks of life
- if you mobilize adequate human and financial resources for the fight
- if you devise and carry out national plans to fight AIDS as an integral part of your health system
- if you ensure the coordinated action of all sectors concerned in your country – education, culture, interior, finance, communications, and the like – by setting up, for example, a central multi-sectoral committee at the highest government level

- if you muster the support of nongovernmental organizations in all the sectors concerned
- if you inspire people to become health promoters to ensure that they, their families, and the communities in which they live behave in such a way as not to become infected with HIV
- if you ensure the understanding and cooperation of people at special risk
- if you make sure that HIV-positive people and AIDS patients are not discriminated against, not ostracized, not stigmatized, not marginalized
- if you pursue vigorous information and education programmes, using all the appropriate media and being very active in educational establishments, starting with those for the young
- if you persuade the media to assume a socially responsible role in informing the public about AIDS and ways of preventing it
- if you train the health professions to inform and educate others and to counsel those infected with HIV, those suffering from AIDS, and their families and friends
- if you educate your health professions to provide those suffering from AIDS and the AIDS-related complex with devoted and humane care
- if you ensure the safety of blood, blood products, and invasive practices on people within and outside the health system
- if you energetically promote suitable education as well as adequate information to ensure the sterility of all syringes, needles, and other instruments used in medical practice as well as other skin-piercing instruments used on people
- if you ensure that the health and social services needed to support and strengthen behaviour change are indeed accessible
- if those of you who are in a position to do so support developing countries in setting up and carrying out national AIDS plans, including information and education that are appropriate to their needs and culture, and in taking measures to strengthen their health infrastructure
- if you insist that the United Nations system and all other development partners coordinate their efforts to ensure synergistic support to your countries
- if you do all of this in line with WHO's global strategy to prevent and control AIDS and in a spirit of worldwide health solidarity
- if you do all this without in any way compromising your commitment to the policies of health for all and primary health care.

Then you can be confident that you *can* and *will* slow the spread of HIV infection, starting now. So let the resolutely determined outcome of this Summit be one of world solidarity in the face of the common enemy AIDS. We can and will stop AIDS. But first of all we will slow the spread of HIV, starting now.

ANNEX 1

London Declaration on AIDS Prevention

28 JANUARY 1988

The World Summit of Ministers of Health on Programmes for AIDS Prevention, involving delegates from 148 countries representing the vast majority of the people of the world, makes the following declaration:

1. Since AIDS is a global problem that poses a serious threat to humanity, urgent action by all governments and people the world over is needed to implement WHO's global AIDS strategy as defined by the Fortieth World Health Assembly and supported by the United Nations General Assembly.

2. We shall do all in our power to ensure that our governments do indeed undertake such urgent action.

3. We undertake to devise national programmes to prevent and contain the spread of human immunodeficiency virus (HIV) infection as part of our countries' health systems. We commend to all governments the value of a high-level coordinating committee to bring together all government sectors, and we shall involve to the fullest extent possible all governmental sectors and relevant nongovernmental organizations in the planning and implementation of such programmes in conformity with the global AIDS strategy.

4. We recognize that, particularly in the absence at present of a vaccine or cure for AIDS, the single most important component of national AIDS programmes is information and education because HIV transmission can be prevented through informed and responsible behaviour. In this respect, individuals, governments, the media and other sectors all have major roles to play in preventing the spread of HIV infection.

5. We consider that information and education programmes should be aimed at the general public and should take full account of social and cultural patterns, different lifestyles, and human and spiritual values. The same principles should apply equally to programmes directed

towards specific groups, involving these groups as appropriate. These include groups such as:

- policy makers
- health and social service workers at all levels
- international travellers
- persons whose practices may place them at increased risk of infection
- the media
- youth and those that work with them, especially teachers
- community and religious leaders
- potential blood donors
- those with HIV infections, their relatives, and others concerned with their care, all of whom need appropriate counselling.

6. We emphasize the need in AIDS prevention programmes to protect human rights and human dignity. Discrimination against, and stigmatization of, HIV-infected people and people with AIDS and population groups undermine public health and must be avoided.

7. We urge the media to fulfil their important social responsibility to provide factual and balanced information to the general public on AIDS and on ways of preventing its spread.

8. We shall seek the involvement of all relevant governmental sectors and nongovernmental organizations in creating the supportive social environment needed to ensure the effective implementation of AIDS prevention programmes and humane care of affected individuals.

9. We shall impress on our governments the importance for national health of ensuring the availability of the human and financial resources, including health and social services with well-trained personnel, needed to carry out our national AIDS programmes and in order to support informed and responsible behaviour.

10. In the spirit of United Nations General Assembly resolution A/42/8, we appeal:

- to all appropriate organizations of the United Nations system, including the specialized agencies
- to bilateral and multilateral agencies
- to nongovernmental and voluntary organizations

to support the worldwide struggle against AIDS in conformity with WHO's global strategy.

11. We appeal in particular to these bodies to provide well-coordinated support to developing countries in setting up and carrying out national AIDS programmes in the light of their needs. We recognize that these needs vary from country to country in the light of their epidemiological situation.

12. We also appeal to those involved in dealing with drug abuse to

intensify their efforts in the spirit of the International Conference on Drug Abuse and Illicit Trafficking (Vienna, June 1987) with a view to contributing to reduction in the spread of HIV infection.

13. We call on the World Health Organization, through its Global Programme on AIDS, to continue to:

  (i) exercise its mandate to direct and coordinate the worldwide effort against AIDS;
 (ii) promote, encourage, and support the worldwide collection and dissemination of accurate information on AIDS;
(iii) develop and issue guidelines on the planning, implementation, monitoring, and evaluation of information and education programmes, including the related research and development, and ensure that these guidelines are updated and revised in the light of evolving experience;
 (iv) support countries in monitoring and evaluating preventive programmes, including information and education activities, and encourage wide dissemination of the findings in order to help countries to learn from the experience of others;
  (v) support and strengthen national programmes for the prevention and control of AIDS.

14. Following from this Summit, 1988 shall be a Year of Communication and Cooperation about AIDS in which we shall:

- open fully the channels of communication in each society so as to inform and educate more widely, broadly, and intensively;
- strengthen the exchange of information and experience among all countries; and
- forge, through information and education and social leadership, a spirit of social tolerance.

15. We are convinced that, by promoting responsible behaviour and through international cooperation, we *can* and *will* begin *now to slow the spread of HIV infection.*

ANNEX 2

AIDS cases reported to WHO as of 20 January 1988

TABLE 1. *AIDS cases reported to WHO by region and country as of 20 January 1988*

African Region		

Country or area	Date of most recent report	Cases reported
Algeria	01/06/1987	5
Angola	26/09/1986	6
Benin	18/05/1987	3
Botswana	10/10/1987	13
Burkina Faso	30/06/1987	26
Burundi	15/10/1987	569
Cameroon	05/03/1987	25
Cape Verde	30/04/1987	4
Central African Republic	31/10/1986	254
Chad	13/11/1986	1
Comoros	13/11/1986	0
Congo	13/11/1986	250
Côte d'Ivoire	20/11/1987	250
Ethiopia	04/12/1987	19
Gabon	06/07/1987	13
Gambia	16/03/1987	14
Ghana	25/05/1987	145
Guinea	12/11/1987	4
Guinea-Bissau	20/11/1987	16
Kenya	10/11/1987	964
Lesotho	27/11/1987	2
Liberia	12/06/1987	2
Madagascar	25/04/1987	0
Malawi	13/11/1986	13
Mali	08/09/1987	0
Mauritania	13/11/1986	0
Mauritius	18/12/1987	1
Mozambique	08/12/1987	4
Niger	14/10/1987	9
Nigeria	22/05/1987	5
Réunion	10/06/1987	1
Rwanda	30/11/1986	705

African Region – *contd.*

Country or area	Date of most recent report	Cases reported
Sao Tome and Principe	01/12/1986	0
Senegal	04/12/1987	66
Seychelles	13/11/1986	0
Sierra Leone	03/11/1987	0
South Africa	04/01/1988	98
Swaziland	01/07/1987	7
Togo	10/12/1987	2
Uganda	31/10/1987	2369
United Republic of Tanzania	17/10/1987	1608
Zaire	30/06/1987	335
Zambia	09/12/1987	536
Zimbabwe	28/08/1987	380
Total		8724

Region of the Americas

Country or area	Date of most recent report	Cases reported
Anguilla	31/03/1987	2
Antigua	30/06/1987	3
Argentina	30/09/1987	120
Bahamas	16/10/1987	163
Barbados	30/09/1987	52
Belize	30/09/1987	4
Bermuda	30/09/1987	75
Bolivia	16/10/1987	4
British Virgin Islands	31/03/1987	0
Brazil	12/07/1987	2325
Canada	07/01/1988	1435
Cayman Islands	31/03/1987	2
Chile	30/09/1987	56
Colombia	30/09/1987	153
Costa Rica	30/09/1987	39
Cuba	16/10/1987	6
Dominica	30/09/1987	5
Dominican Republic	30/09/1987	352
Ecuador	30/09/1987	52
El Salvador	03/10/1987	16
French Guiana	30/09/1987	93
Grenada	30/09/1987	7
Guadeloupe	30/06/1987	51
Guatemala	30/09/1987	30
Guyana	30/09/1987	5
Haiti	30/09/1987	912
Honduras	15/09/1987	51
Jamaica	30/09/1987	30
Martinique	30/06/1987	27
Mexico	16/10/1987	713
Montserrat	30/09/1987	0
Nicaragua	18/09/1987	19
Panama	30/09/1987	22

Paraguay	30/06/1987	14
Peru	30/09/1987	44
Saint Kitts and Nevis	30/09/1987	1
Saint Lucia	30/09/1987	6
Saint Vincent	30/09/1987	7
Suriname	30/09/1987	6
Trinidad and Tobago	30/11/1987	206
Turks and Caicos	30/06/1987	4
United States of America	28/12/1987	49743
Uruguay	30/09/1987	14
Venezuela	30/09/1987	101
Total		56970

South-East Asia Region

Country or area	Date of most recent report	Cases reported
Bangladesh	14/04/1987	0
Bhutan	14/04/1987	0
Burma	14/04/1987	0
Democratic People's Republic of Korea	09/05/1987	0
India	09/05/1987	9
Indonesia	21/04/1987	1
Maldives	30/06/1987	0
Mongolia	31/12/1987	0
Nepal	09/05/1987	0
Sri Lanka	14/04/1987	2
Thailand	12/10/1987	12
Total		24

European Region

Country or area	Date of most recent report	Cases reported
Albania	31/08/1987	0
Austria	30/09/1987	120
Belgium	30/09/1987	280
Bulgaria	06/10/1987	3
Czechoslovakia	31/03/1987	7
Denmark	30/09/1987	202
Finland	30/09/1987	22
France	30/09/1987	2523
German Democratic Republic	30/06/1987	4
Germany, Federal Republic of	31/12/1987	1669
Greece	30/09/1987	78
Hungary	30/09/1987	6
Iceland	30/09/1987	4
Ireland	30/09/1987	25
Israel	30/09/1987	43
Italy	30/09/1987	1104
Luxembourg	30/09/1987	8
Malta	30/09/1987	7

European Region – *contd.*

Country or area	Date of most recent report	Cases reported
Netherlands	30/09/1987	370
Norway	30/09/1887	64
Poland	30/06/1987	3
Portugal	30/09/1987	81
Romania	31/03/1987	2
Spain	30/09/1987	624
Sweden	07/12/1987	156
Switzerland	30/09/1987	299
Turkey	30/06/1987	21
United Kingdom	04/12/1987	1170
USSR	05/08/1987	4
Yugoslavia	30/09/1987	21
Total		8920

Eastern Mediterranean Region

Country or area	Date of most recent report	Cases reported
Cyprus	01/06/1987	3
Djibouti	01/10/1987	0
Egypt	06/07/1987	1
Jordan	24/12/1987	3
Lebanon	03/06/1987	3
Qatar	09/05/1987	9
Sudan	23/08/1987	12
Tunisia	06/12/1987	11
Other countries	10/09/1987	36
Total		78

Western Pacific Region

Country or area	Date of most recent report	Cases reported
Australia	07/12/1987	681
Brunei Darussalam	08/09/1987	0
China (Mainland)	08/09/1987	2
China (Province of Taiwan)	26/01/1986	1
Cook Islands	08/09/1987	0
Fiji	08/09/1987	0
French Polynesia	08/09/1987	1
Hong Kong	17/11/1987	6
Japan	14/12/1987	59
Kiribati	26/10/1987	0
Malaysia	08/09/1987	1
Mariana Islands	05/08/1987	0
New Caledonia	08/09/1987	0
New Zealand	14/12/1987	59

Papua New Guinea	08/09/1987	0
Philippines	30/10/1987	10
Republic of Korea	08/09/1987	1
Samoa	08/09/1987	0
Singapore	30/06/1987	2
Solomon Islands	08/09/1987	0
Tonga	06/10/1987	1
Tuvalu	08/09/1987	0
Vanuatu	08/09/1987	0
Viet Nam	08/09/1987	0
Total		824

TABLE 2. *AIDS cases reported to WHO by year as of 20/01/1988*

Continent	Pre-1979	1979	1980	1981	1982	1983	1984	1985	1986	1987	1988	Total
Africa	1	0	0	0	3	14	82	206	2441	6001	0	8748
Americas	68	14	66	277	1054	3188	6267	11302	17090	17644	0	56970
Asia	0	0	1	0	1	8	4	29	54	127	0	224
Europe	5	0	3	16	72	219	576	1389	2641	3935	0	8856
Oceania	0	0	0	0	2	6	45	124	240	325	0	742
Total	74	14	70	293	1132	3435	6974	13050	22466	28032	0	75540

TABLE 3. *Cumulative AIDS cases after 1979 reported to WHO by year as of 20/01/1988*

Continent	Pre-1979	1979	1980	1981	1982	1983	1984	1985	1986	1987	1988	Total
Africa	1	0	0	0	3	17	99	305	2746	8747	8747	8748
Americas	68	14	80	357	1411	4599	10866	22168	39258	56902	56902	56970
Asia	0	0	1	1	2	10	14	43	97	224	224	224
Europe	5	0	3	19	91	310	886	2275	4916	8851	8851	8856
Oceania	0	0	0	0	2	8	53	177	417	742	742	742
Total	74	14	84	377	1509	4944	11918	24968	47434	75466	75466	75540

TABLE 4. *Cases reported by continent as of 20/01/1988*

Continent	Number of cases	Number of countries or territories reporting		
		to WHO	0 cases	1 or more cases
Africa	8748	48	8	40
Americas	56970	44	2	42
Asia	224	28	9	19
Europe	8856	28	1	27
Oceania	742	14	10	4
Total	75540	162	30	132

TABLE 5. *Cases reported by WHO region as of 20/01/1988*

| WHO Region | Number of cases | Number of countries or territories reporting | | |
		to WHO	0 cases	1 or more cases
Africa	8724	44	7	37
Americas	56970	44	2	42
South-East Asia	24	11	7	4
Europe	8920	30	1	29
Eastern Mediterranean	78	9	1	8
Western Pacific	824	24	12	12
Total	75540	162	30	132

Social Aspects of AIDS Prevention and Control Programmes*

The Global Programme on AIDS of the World Health Organization has worked with national authorities in developing over 100 national programmes for the prevention and control of AIDS throughout the world. While these national programmes operate in substantially different epidemiological, social, economic and political cnvironments, they have been faced with a similar range of complex social issues, involving such areas as screening, employment, housing, access to health care and schooling. In the light of the experience of these national programmes to date, as well as current knowledge about human immunodeficiency virus (HIV) infection and AIDS, the Global Programme on AIDS wishes to draw attention, through this statement, to the following social aspects of AIDS prevention and control.

1. AIDS prevention and control strategies can be implemented effectively and efficiently and evaluated in a manner that respects and protects human rights.

2. There is no public health rationale to justify isolation, quarantine, or any discriminatory measures based solely on the fact that a person is suspected or known to be infected with HIV. The modes of HIV transmission are limited (sex, blood, mother-to-child) and HIV spreads almost entirely through identifiable behaviours and specific actions which are subject to individual control. In most instances, the active participation of *two* people is required for HIV transmission, such as in sexual intercourse and in sharing contaminated needles or syringes. However, spread of HIV can also be prevented through the health system (e.g., by ensuring the safety of blood, blood products, artificial insemination and organ transplantation, and preventing reuse of

---

* This statement may be updated by the WHO Global Programme on AIDS, on the basis of experience in AIDS prevention and control programmes worldwide, and as additional knowledge about HIV infection and AIDS becomes available.

needles, syringes and other skin-piercing or invasive equipment without proper sterilization).

HIV infection is *not* spread through casual contact, routine social contact in schools, the workplace or public places, nor through water or food, eating utensils, coughing or sneezing, insects, toilets or swimming pools.

Accordingly, an AIDS prevention and control strategy should include:

- **provision of information and education** to the general public, to persons with behaviours that place them at risk of HIV infection (risk behaviour groups), and to HIV-infected persons;
- **counselling** of HIV-infected persons;
- **ensuring the safety** of blood and blood products, skin-piercing practices and other invasive procedures.

In accordance with this strategy, persons suspected or known to be HIV-infected should remain integrated within society to the maximum possible extent and be helped to assume responsibility for preventing HIV transmission to others. Exclusion of persons suspected or known to be HIV-infected would be unjustified in public health terms and would seriously jeopardize educational and other efforts to prevent the spread of HIV. Furthermore, discriminatory measures create additional problems and cause unnecessary human suffering. **The avoidance of discrimination against persons known or suspected to be HIV-infected is important for AIDS prevention and control; failure to prevent such discrimination may endanger public health.**

3. Determination of an individual's HIV-infection status may occur through medical examination for suspected HIV-related illness, voluntary testing programmes, screening of blood donors, or in other settings. Testing for the purpose of determining an individual's HIV-infection status should involve informed consent and counselling and should ensure confidentiality.

The Global Programme on AIDS has already laid down criteria for HIV-screening programmes* which emphasize the need to consider carefully the public health rationale for such screening as well as to address explicitly the technical, operational, economic, social, legal and ethical issues inherent in screening programmes (see Annex 4).

---

* *Report of the Meeting on Criteria for HIV-Screening Programmes, Geneva, 20–21 May 1987.* Unpublished WHO document WHO/SPA/GLO/87.2

ANNEX 4

Screening and Testing in AIDS Prevention and Control Programmes

Screening is the examination of entire populations or groups within populations to determine their infection or disease status.

Testing is the determination of infection or disease status for an individual.

The Global Programme on AIDS has worked with national authorities in over 100 countries to develop programmes for AIDS prevention and control. In this context, screening for human immunodeficiency virus (HIV) infection has often been discussed to determine its role, if any, in national AIDS programmes. HIV screening involves many complex technical, logistical, social, legal and ethical issues; to help ensure their complete analysis and review, the Programme convened a meeting of health experts on screening for HIV infection.* The meeting listed a broad range of issues that must be considered, including:

1 the rationale of the proposed programme;
2 the population to be screened;
3 the test method to be used;
4 where the laboratory testing is to be done;
5 the intended use of data obtained from testing;
6 the plan for communicating results to the person tested;
7 how counselling is to be accomplished;
8 the social impact of screening;
9 legal and ethical considerations raised by the proposed screening programme.

---

* Single copies of the *Report of the Meeting on Criteria for HIV Screening Programmes, Geneva, 20–21 May 1987 (WHO/SPA/GLO/87.2)* can be obtained from the Global Programme on AIDS, WHO, Avenue Appia, CH-1211 Geneva 27, Switzerland.

In the light of:

- the Report of the Meeting of Experts;
- the experience of national programmes to date;
- current knowledge about HIV infection and AIDS;

the **World Health Organization Global Programme on AIDS** wishes to draw attention to the following issues related to screening and testing in AIDS prevention and control programmes.

1 **Screening programmes** for HIV infection can help:
- prevent transmission through blood supplies, semen, tissues, or organs for transplant;
- obtain epidemiological information on HIV prevalence or incidence.

2 **Whenever a screening programme** is under consideration, all the issues raised by the expert meeting should be explicitly addressed and resolved. Poorly designed or implemented HIV-screening programmes will be detrimental to public health, and will waste resources. Public health needs and human rights will be best served by carefully considering the entire range of technical, logistical, social, legal and ethical issues **before** deciding whether to proceed with any screening programme.

3 **Mandatory screening** for HIV has only a very limited role in programmes for AIDS prevention and control. Mandatory screening of donors is useful to prevent HIV transmission through blood, semen, or other cells, tissues or organs. This screening should involve informed consent and counselling and should ensure confidentiality.

4 **Serosurveys** help clarify the epidemiological pattern of HIV, which is useful to assess the areas and groups that need specific educational programmes or other preventive services. These surveys can be conducted using methods that do not threaten human rights. Such surveys can either involve informed consent and counselling and ensure confidentiality or they may be anonymous (no record of name or other specific identifiers).

5 **Voluntary HIV testing** may form part of medical care for suspected HIV-related illness and may also be provided as a service to individuals in conjunction with information and education, counselling and other support services to help promote sustained behaviour change. Voluntary HIV testing should involve informed consent and counselling and should ensure confidentiality.

6 **Voluntary HIV testing services** should be made widely available as part of AIDS prevention and control programmes, and access to such services should be facilitated.

List of Participants*

* This list was compiled by the Department of Health and Social Security, United Kingdom. An asterisk denotes a delegate who spoke at the Summit, and whose speech is available from: Global Programme on AIDS, World Health Organization, 1211 Geneva 27, Switzerland.

Governmental Delegations

AFGHANISTAN

Head of Delegation
Dr H. S. Bahador
Minister of Health

Delegates
Dr D. Habib
Head, International Department,
  Ministry of Public Health

Mr A. Sarwar
Chargé d'Affaires, Embassy of the
  Republic of Afghanistan, London

ALGERIA

Head of Delegation
Mr D. Houhou
Minister of Health

Delegates
Professor A. Bouguermouh
Co-ordinator, Committee on Sexually
  Transmitted Diseases and AIDS

Professor B. Ait Ouyahia
Director-General, National Institute of
  Public Health

Mr M. Boukari
Cultural Counsellor, Embassy of the
  People's Democratic Republic of
  Algeria, London

ANGOLA

Head of Delegation
Dr A. J. Ferreira Neto
Minister of Health

Delegates
Dr J. Leite Da Costa

Dr T. M. Da Soledade Silva Alves Faria
Embassy of the People's Republic of
  Angola, London

ANTIGUA and BARBUDA

Head of Delegation
Mr A. E. Freeland
Minister of Labour, Health and Co-
  operatives

Delegates
Dr T. Jones
Chief Medical Officer, Ministry of
  Health

Miss I. V. Wallace
Superintendent of Public Health
  Nursing/Supervisor of Health
  Education
Ministry of Health

ARGENTINA

Head of Delegation
Dr R. Rodriguez
Secretary of State for Health

Delegate
Mr J. E. Fleming

AUSTRALIA

Head of Delegation
Dr N. Blewett
Minister for Community Affairs and
  Health

Delegates
Professor A. Basten
Chairman, AIDS Task Force

Professor R. Penny

Chairman, National Advisory
  Committee on AIDS

Miss D. Snow
Senior Private Secretary to Minister

Dr D. Steel
Counsellor, Australian High
  Commission, London

Mr I. Haupt
Officer, Department of Community
  Services and Health

AUSTRIA

Head of Delegation
Dr G. Liebeswar
Director-General of Public Health

BAHAMAS

Head of Delegation
Dr N. R. Gay
Minister of Health

Delegate
Dr P. Gomez
Specialist in Infectious Diseases

BAHRAIN

Head of Delegation
Mr J. S. Al-Arrayed
Minister of Health

Delegates
Dr R. Fulayfil
Under-Secretary and Chairman of AIDS
  Committee, Ministry of Health

Dr K. Al-Arrayed
Deputy Chief Medical Staff, Salmaniya
  Medical Centre

Dr M. Al-Khateeb
Director of Public Health Education,
  Ministry of Health

BANGLADESH

Head of Delegation
Professor N. Islam
Chairman, National AIDS Committee

Delegates
Professor N. Islam
Associate Professor of Virology and
Secretary National AIDS Committee for
  the People's Republic of Bangladesh

Mr S. A. Jalal
Counsellor, Bangladesh High
  Commission, London

BARBADOS

Head of Delegation
Mr M. Taitt*
Minister of Health

Delegates
Mrs A. Haynes
Deputy Permanent Secretary, Ministry
  of Health

Professor E. R. Walrond
Chairman, National Advisory
  Committee on AIDS

BELGIUM

Head of Delegation
Mrs W. Demeester-De Meyer
Secretary of State for Public Health and
  Policy on Disability

Delegates
Dr J. Desmyter
Chairman, National AIDS Committee

Dr A. Stroobant
Adviser to the Minister

BELIZE

Head of Delegation
Dr J. Alpuche*
Minister of Health

Delegates
Dr J. A. Lopez
Epidemiologist

Mr A. A. Woodye
First Secretary, Belize High
  Commission, London

BENIN

Head of Delegation

Dr H. Sanoussi*
Director-General, Ministry of Health

Delegate

Dr S. I. Zohoun
Permanent Secretary, National AIDS
  Committee

BHUTAN

Head of Delegation

Dr T. Yountan
Director-General of Health Services
Ministry of Social Services

Delegate

Dr S. Thinley
Specialist in Dermatology
Thimphu General Hospital

BOLIVIA

Dr L. Camacho
Adviser to the Minister of Health

BOTSWANA

Head of Delegation

Dr J. L. T. Mothibamele*
Minister of Health

Delegate

Dr E. T. Maganu
Director of Health Services, Ministry of
  Health

BRAZIL

Head of Delegation

Dr L. Borges Da Silveira
Minister of Health

Delegates

Mr R. Malcotti
Head of International Health Affairs
  Office
Ministry of Health

Dr L. Guerra de Macedo Rodrigues
Director, National Division of Sexually
  Transmitted Diseases and AIDS
Ministry of Health

Mr L. H. Sobreira Lopes
Second Secretary, Brazilian Embassy,
  London

BULGARIA

Head of Delegation

Professor L. Shindarov*
First Deputy Minister of Health and
  Social Welfare

Delegates

Professor P. I. Vachkov
Head of Department, Medical Academy
National Co-ordinator on AIDS

Mr A. Peytchev
First Secretary, Bulgarian Embassy,
  London

BURKINA FASO

Head of Delegation

Dr A. D. Sougba
Minister of Health and Social Services

Delegate

Dr H. Tiendrebeogo
Secretary General
Ministry of Health and Social Services

BURMA

Head of Delegation

Dr Tun Hla Pru*
Deputy Minister of Health

Delegate

Dr U. Aye Nyein
Lecturer/Dermatologist/Venereologist
Rangoon General Hospital

BURUNDI

Head of Delegation

Dr T. Niyunguka
Minister of Public Health

Delegate

Dr D. Seruzingo
General Inspector for Public Health,
  Ministry of Public Health

CANADA

Head of Delegation
Mr J. Epp*
Minister of National Health and Welfare

Delegates
Dr M. Law
Deputy Minister of National Health and
  Welfare

Mr I. Shugart
Senior Policy Adviser to the Minister

Dr A. J. Clayton
Director-General, Federal Centre for
  AIDS

Dr N. Gilmore
Chairman, National Advisory
  Committee on AIDS

CAPE VERDE

Head of Delegation
Dr I. F. Gomes*
Minister of Health

Delegates
Dr D. P. Andrade
Director of AIDS Programme

Dr D. Dantas Dos Reis
Clinical Director, Agostinho Neto
  Hospital

CENTRAL AFRICAN REPUBLIC

Head of Delegation
Mr J. Willybiro-Sako
Minister of Health and Social Welfare

Delegate
Professor M. D. Vohito
Chairman, AIDS Committee

CHAD

Head of Delegation
Dr Y. P. Matchock Mahouri*
Director-General of Public Health,
  Ministry of Public Health

Delegate
Dr H. M. Hassan
Director of Primary Health Care

CHILE

Dr J. M. Pertuze
Representative of the Minister of Health

CHINA

Head of Delegation
Dr Wang Shusheng
Chief, Antiepidemic Station of Guangxi

COLOMBIA

Head of Delegation
Dr R. Samper
Chargé d'Affaires, Embassy of
  Colombia, London

COMOROS

Head of Delegation
Mr A. Hassanali
Minister of Public Health and
  Population

Delegate
Dr M. Velo
Director of Public Health Programmes
Ministry of Public Health and
  Population

CONGO

Head of Delegation
Mr B. Combo-Matsiona*
Minister of Health and Social Affairs

Delegates
Dr P. Mpele
General Secretary, National AIDS
  Programme

Mr L. Muzzu
Honorary Consul, Embassy of the
  People's Republic of the Congo,
  London

COSTA RICA

Professor L. J. Mata
Chairman, National AIDS Committee

COTE D'IVOIRE

Head of Delegation

Professor M. A. Djedje*
Minister of Public Health and
  Population

Delegate

Professor K. P. Odehouri
Chairman, National Committee against
  AIDS

CUBA

Head of Delegation

Dr H. J. T. Molinert
Deputy Minister, Ministry of Public
  Health

Delegates

Mr J. Heredia, First Secretary,
  Permanent Mission of the Republic of
  Cuba to the United Nations Office and
  other International Organizations at
  Geneva

Mr F. A. Machado Ramirez
Director, AIDS Research Laboratory

CYPRUS

Head of Delegation

Mr H. Hadjipanayiotou
Director-General, Ministry of Health

Delegate

Dr M. Voniatis
Senior Medical Officer, Ministry of
  Health

CZECHOSLOVAKIA

Head of Delegation

Professor J. Prokopec
Minister of Health of the Czech Socialist
  Republic

Delegates

Dr I. Masar
Deputy Director, Public Health
  Services, Ministry of Health of the
  Slovak Socialist Republic

Professor J. Sejda
Chief, Epidemiology Department,

Postgraduate Medical Institute,
  Prague

Mr Z. Tula
Foreign Relations Department, Ministry
  of Health of the Czech Socialist
  Republic

DEMOCRATIC YEMEN

Head of Delegation

Dr S. Sharaf
Minister of Public Health

Delegates

Dr F. M. Kaid
Chairman, National AIDS Committee

Mr M. A. Zokari
Economic Counsellor, Embassy of the
  People's Democratic Republic of
  Yemen, London

DENMARK

Head of Delegation

Mrs A. Laustsen*
Minister of Health

Delegates

Mrs J. Mersing
Deputy Permanent Secretary, Ministry
  of Health

Dr S. K. Sorensen
Director-General, National Board of
  Health

Mr E. Svenningsen
Deputy Director, Ministry of Foreign
  Affairs

Miss H. Nielsen
Deputy Chief of Section, Danish
  International Development Agency
  (DANIDA)

DJIBOUTI

Head of Delegation

Mr H. I. Ougoure*
Minister of Public Health and Social
  Affairs

Delegates

Dr S. S. Youssouf
Assistant Director, Public Health
  Department

Professor J. P. Albert
Technical Adviser, Ministry of Public
  Health and Social Affairs

DOMINICA

Head of Delegation

Mr R. A. David*
Minister of Health

Delegate

Dr W. E. V. Green
Medical Officer and Chairman, AIDS
  Task Force, Ministry of Health

DOMINICAN REPUBLIC

Head of Delegation

Dr R. Tallaj*
Deputy Minister of Health

Delegates

Dr E. Guerror
Director of Sexually Transmitted
  Diseases and AIDS Programme

Dr I. Hernandez
Viral Epidemiologist, AIDS Programme

ECUADOR

Head of Delegation

Mr R. Perez y Reyna
Ambassador of Ecuador, London

Delegates

Dr A. Maldonado Mejia
Technical Assistant, Ministry of Health

Mrs H. Martinez de Perez
Minister, Embassy of Ecuador, London

Mr R. Paredes
Second Secretary, Embassy of Ecuador,
  London

EGYPT

Head of Delegation

Dr M. R. Dewidar*
Minister of Health

Delegates

Professor Y. El Battawy
Dean, Faculty of Medicine, Cairo
  University

Dr M. Fansa
Medical Counsellor, Embassy of the
  Arab Republic of Egypt, London

Dr H. Koura
Medical Attaché, Embassy of the Arab
  Republic of Egypt, London

EL SALVADOR

Dr R. G. Villacorta
Deputy Minister of Public Health and
  Social Welfare

EQUATORIAL GUINEA

Head of Delegation

Mr M. Nsoro Mbana
Minister of Health

Delegate

Dr J. Ntutumu Nsue
Head of Epidemiology Services,
  Ministry of Health

ETHIOPIA

Head of Delegation

Dr G. Tsehay*
Minister of Health

Delegate

Dr G. Gizaw
Head of AIDS Prevention and Control
  Programme, Ministry of Health

FINLAND

Head of Delegation

Mrs A. H. Pesola*
Minister for Social Affairs and Health

Delegates

Dr H. Hellberg
Chairman, National AIDS Committee

Dr M. Murtomaa
Director, National Board of Health

Mrs L. Ollila
Secretary for International Affairs,
  Ministry of Social Affairs and Health

FRANCE

Head of Delegation

Dr M. Barzach
Minister of Health and the Family

Delegates

Professor J. F. Girard
Director-General of Health, Ministry of
  Social Affairs and Employment

Professor A. Pompidou
Co-ordinator, National AIDS
  Programme

Dr H. Rossert
Technical Adviser, French Committee
  for Health Education

Dr F. Varet
International Relations Division,
  Ministry of Social Affairs and
  Employment

Mrs F. Nicoliai
Press Attaché, French Committee for
  Health Education

Mrs J. Chauvet
Counsellor (Social Affairs), French
  Embassy, London

Mrs P. Daix
Press Attaché

GABON

Head of Delegation

Dr J. P. Okias
Minister of Public Health and
  Population

Delegates

Mr C. M. Diop
Ambassador of the Republic of Gabon,
  London

Dr G. E. Roenants
Director-General, International Centre
  for Medical Research

GAMBIA

Head of Delegation

Mrs L. A. Njie
Minister of Health, Environment,
  Labour and Social Welfare

Delegates

Dr H. A. B. Njie
Director of Medical Services and
  Chairman of AIDS Committee

Mr S. Cessay
Health Education Officer

GERMAN DEMOCRATIC REPUBLIC

Head of Delegation

Professor L. Mecklinger*
Minister of Health

Delegates

Professor S. Dittmann
Director, GDR Central Institute of
  Hygiene, Microbiology and
  Epidemiology

Mr M. Rudolph
First Secretary, Embassy of the German
  Democratic Republic, London

GERMANY, FEDERAL REPUBLIC OF

Head of Delegation

Professor R. Sussmuth
Federal Minister of Youth, Family
  Affairs, Women and Health

Delegates

Professor M. Steinbach
Director-General, Federal Ministry for
  Youth, Family Affairs, Women and
  Health

Dr X. Scheil-Adlung
Head of Division, Federal Ministry for
  Youth, Family Affairs, Women and
  Health

Dr W. Hoffman
First Counsellor, Scientific Affairs,
  Embassy of the Federal Republic of
  Germany, London

Mr H. Braun
First Secretary, Press and Public Affairs,
  Embassy of the Federal Republic of
  Germany, London

Mrs Fremerey
Head of Press Section, Federal Ministry
  of Youth, Family Affairs, Women and
  Health

GHANA

Head of Delegation
Mr F. W. K. Klutse
Secretary for Health

Delegates
Dr M. Adibo
Director of Medical Services

Dr A. Neequaye
Chairman, Technical Committee on
  AIDS

Mr Y. O. Osei
First Secretary, Ghana High
  Commission, London

GREECE

Head of Delegation
Mr G. Solomos
Minister of Health and Social Welfare

Delegates
Professor G. Papaevangelou
Chairman, National AIDS Committee

Miss I. Vasilopoulou
Minister's Office

GRENADA

Head of Delegation
Mr D. Williams*
Minister of Health and Housing

Delegate
Mr O. M. Gibbs
High Commissioner, London

GUATEMALA

Head of Delegation
Dr C. A. Soto Gomez
Minister of Public Health and Social
  Welfare

Delegate
Dr E. Blandon
Ambassador of Guatemala, London

GUINEA

Head of Delegation
Dr M. P. Diallo*
Minister of Health and Social Affairs

Delegate
Dr K. Kourouma
Co-ordinator, Sexually Transmitted
  Diseases and AIDS Committee

GUINEA-BISSAU

Head of Delegation
Mr A. Nunes Correia
Minister of Public Health

Delegate
Dr A. P. J. da Silva
Director, National AIDS Programme

GUYANA

Mr C. J. E. Barker
Acting High Commissioner, London

HAITI

Head of Delegation
Dr J. M. Verly
Minister of Public Health and
  Population

Delegate
Dr L. Eustache
Chief Co-ordinator, National AIDS
  Commission

HOLY SEE

Head of Delegation
Archbishop F. Angelini

Delegates
Dr P. Linehan
Sister M. M. Lawlor

HONDURAS

Head of Delegation
Dr R. A. Villeda-Bermudez*
Minister of Health

Delegates

Mr J. D. Villatoro-Hall
Minister-Counsellor, Embassy of
  Honduras, London

Dr J. E. Zelaya
Head of Epidemiology Division,
  Ministry of Health
  and Co-ordinator, National AIDS
  Commission

HUNGARY

Head of Delegation

Dr L. Medve
Secretary of State, Ministry of Social
  Affairs and Health

Delegates

Professor Z. Hollin
Director, National Trust for
  Haematology and Blood Transfusion

Dr M. Kökény
Special Adviser, Council of Ministers

Mr M. Orban
Scientific and Technical Secretary
Embassy of the Hungarian People's
  Republic, London

ICELAND

Head of Delegation

Mr G. Bjarnason*
Minister of Health and Social Security

Delegates

Dr P. Sigurdsson
Secretary-General, Ministry of Health
  and Social Security

Dr O. Olafsson
Director-General of Health and Social
  Security

INDIA

Head of Delegation

Mr P. V. Narasimha Rao*
Minister of Health and Welfare

Delegates

Mr S. S. Dhanoa
Secretary, Ministry of Health and Family
  Welfare

Mr S. N. Rao

Counsellor, Indian High Commission,
  London

Mr R. P. Watal
Private Secretary to the Minister of
  Health and Family Welfare

INDONESIA

Head of Delegation

Dr S. Surjaningrat
Minister of Health

Delegates

Mr S. L. Leimena
Director-General for Prevention and
  Eradication of Contagious Diseases

Dr W. B. Wanandi
Technical Adviser to the Minister of
  Health

Mrs T. Suyono
Counsellor, Head of Information,
  Indonesian Embassy, London

IRAQ

Head of Delegation

Dr S. H. Alwash*
Minister of Health

Delegates

Dr T. Hilail Al-Ani
Consultant Dermatologist and
  Venereologist, City Teaching
  Hospital, Baghdad

Dr M. Al-Najjar
Director-General of Health Relations,
  Ministry of Health

Dr Z. Kassir
Professor of Medicine, University of
  Baghdad

Dr M. M. S. Mahood
Department of Preventive Medicine,
  Ministry of Health

IRELAND

Head of Delegation

Dr R. O'Hanlon
Minister of Health

Delegates

Dr J. H. Walsh
Deputy Chief Medical Officer,
  Department of Health

Mr P. W. Flanagan
Permanent Secretary

Mr B. O'Reilly
Third Secretary, Irish Embassy, London

Mr A. Smith
Private Secretary to the Minister of
  Health

ISRAEL

Head of Delegation

Professor A. Morag*
Chairman, Sub-Committee on AIDS
  Information

Delegates

Mrs Y. Rubinstein
Second Secretary, Embassy of Israel,
  London

Mr I. Shenker
AIDS Education, Hadash Hospital

ITALY

Head of Delegation

Dr M. Caponetto
Principal Private Secretary to Minister of
  Health

Delegates

Professor M. Colombini
Director of International Relations,
  Ministry of Health

Mrs R. Corui
Director, Nursing School, "Gemelli"
  Teaching Hospital

Professor D. Greco
Director, Higher Institute of Health

Mr M. Fugazzola
Press Counsellor, Italian Embassy,
  London

Dr A. Luna
Chairman, Commission of Information
  on AIDS

Dr G. C. Muslello

International Relations Officer, Ministry
  of Health

Dr E. Rocco
Deputy Director of International
  Relations, Ministry of Health

Professor C. Vetere
Director of Social Medicine, Ministry of
  Health

JAMAICA

Head of Delegation

Dr K. L. Baugh*
Minister of Health

Delegates

Dr J. Lagrende
Chief Medical Officer, Ministry of
  Health

Mrs P. Saunders
Jamaican High Commission, London

JAPAN

Head of Delegation

Mr S. Nagano
Vice-Minister of Health and Welfare

Delegates

Dr M. Ito*
Director of Communicable Diseases
  Control, Ministry of Health and
  Welfare

Mr T. Ito
Counsellor, Embassy of Japan, London

Dr M. Mugitani
Deputy Director, International Affairs
  Division,
Ministry of Health and Welfare

Mr S. Higuchi
First Secretary, Embassy of Japan,
  London

Mr N. Ito
Third Secretary, Embassy of Japan,
  London

JORDAN

Head of Delegation

Dr Z. Hamzeh*
Minister of Health

Delegate
Dr J. Merza
Head, Central Blood Bank

KENYA

Head of Delegation
Mr K. S. N. Matiba
Minister of Health

Delegates
Dr S. Kosgei
High Commissioner, London

Dr F. M. Mueke
AIDS Programme Co-ordinator

Mrs E. N. Ngugi
Lecturer, University of Nairobi College
  of Health Science

Mr K. M. M'Agere
Press Attaché, Kenya High Commission,
  London

Miss S. F. Atandi
Third Secretary, Kenya High
  Commission, London

KIRIBATI

Head of Delegation
Mr R. Ataia
Minister of Health and Family Planning

Delegate
Dr T. Taitai
Chief Medical Officer

KUWAIT

Head of Delegation
Dr A. R. Al-Awadi
Minister of Public Health

Delegates
Dr R. Al-Owashi
Director of Public Health, Ministry of
  Public Health

Dr A. Y. A. Al-Saif
Assistant Under-Secretary for Public
  Affairs, Ministry of Public Health

Professor D. M. K. Behbehani

Chairman, AIDS Committee
Mr Y. Abu-Al-Fottouh
Legal Adviser, Ministry of Public Health

LAO PEOPLE'S DEMOCRATIC REPUBLIC

Head of Delegation
Dr K. Pholsena*
Minister of Public Health

Delegate
Dr B. Mixap
Director, Institute of Hygiene and
  Epidemiology

LEBANON

Dr M. G. Nasser
Representative of Minister of Health

LESOTHO

Head of Delegation
Dr S. T. Makenete
Minister of Health

Delegate
Dr N. C. Moji
Acting Director of Health Services,
  Ministry of Health

LIBERIA

Head of Delegation
Mrs M. S. Belleh*
Minister of Health and Social Welfare

Delegates
Mr N. Davies
Counsellor, Embassy of the Republic of
  Liberia, London

Dr R. A. Peal
Chief of Technical Committee, National
  Advisory Committee on AIDS

LIBYAN ARAB JAMAHIRIYA

Dr E. Elnageh
Head of National AIDS Committee

LUXEMBOURG

Head of Delegation
Dr J. Kohl*
Director of Health, Ministry of Health

Delegates
Dr D. Hansen-Koenig
Deputy Director of Health, Ministry of Health

Dr R. Hemmer
Head of National AIDS Committee

MADAGASCAR

Head of Delegation
Dr J. J. Seraphin
Minister of Health

Delegate
Dr Rasamindrakotroka
Biologist

MALAWI

Head of Delegation
Mr E. C. I. Bwanali*
Minister of Health

Delegate
Dr J. A. Kalilani
Deputy Chief Medical Officer, Ministry of Health

MALAYSIA

Head of Delegation
Dr Chan Siang Sun
Minister of Health

Delegates
Dr A. A. Rahman
Director-General of Health, Ministry of Health

Dr H. R. H. Rahmat
Assistant Director of Health, Ministry of Health

MALDIVES

Head of Delegation
Mr A. Jameel
Minister of Health

Delegate
Dr A. S. Abdullah
Director-General of Health Services, Ministry of Health

MALI

Head of Delegation
Mrs A. Sidibe*
Minister of Public Health and Social Affairs

Delegates
Dr A. Guindo
Chairman, AIDS Committee

Dr Z. Maiga
Technical Adviser to Minister

MALTA

Head of Delegation
Dr L. Galea*
Minister for Social Policy

Delegates
Dr G. Galea
Health Education Unit, Department of Health

Dr A. Vassallo
Principal Medical Officer, Department of Health

Dr C. G. Vella
Adviser for Social Policy, Ministry of Social Policy

Mr G. Naudi
Private Secretary to Minister

MAURITANIA

Dr C. Moctar
Director of Hygiene and Health Protection
Ministry of Health and Social Affairs

MAURITIUS

Head of Delegation
Mr J. Goburdhun
Minister of Health

Delegates
Mr S. Soobiah
High Commissioner, Mauritius High
  Commission, London
Dr P. C. Chan-Kam
Consultant (Dermatology), National
  AIDS Programme Co-ordinator

MEXICO
Head of Delegation
Professor G. Soberón Acevedo*
Secretary of Health
Delegates
Dr J. Kumate Rodriguez
Under-Secretary of Health, Ministry of
  Health
Dr J. Sepulveda
Director-General of Epidemiology,
  Ministry of Health

MONACO
Head of Delegation
Mr D. L. Gastaud
Director, Health and Social Action,
  Ministry of State
Delegate
Dr M. Landy-Verneret
Médecin Inspecteur

MONGOLIA
Head of Delegation
Mr C. H. Tserennadmid*
Minister of Public Health
Delegate
Dr Z. Jadamba
Chief, International Relations
  Department, Ministry of Public
  Health

MOROCCO
Head of Delegation
Mr T. Bencheikh
Minister of Public Health
Delegate
Dr N. Fikri-Benbrahim
Chief, Epidemiology Division, Ministry
  of Health

MOZAMBIQUE
Head of Delegation
Professor F. Vaz
Minister of Health
Delegate
Dr R. G. Vaz
Director of Health, Ministry of Health

NAURU
Head of Delegation
Mr M. Weston
Representative of Nauru in the United
  Kingdom
Delegate
Mrs M. Howard
Personal Assistant

NEPAL
Head of Delegation
Mr G. P. Singh*
Minister of Health
Delegate
Dr V. L. Gurubacharya
National Focal Point for AIDS
  Programme

NETHERLANDS
Head of Delegation
Mr D. J. D. Dees
State Secretary of Welfare, Health and
  Cultural Affairs
Delegates
Mr H. J. Smid
Head, Disease Control Department,
  Ministry of Welfare, Health and
  Cultural Affairs
Mr F. H. de Man
Deputy Head, International Health
  Affairs Division, Ministry of Welfare,
  Health and Cultural Affairs
Professor E. W. Roscam Abbing
Chairman, AIDS Committee
Mr H. W. van de Bie
Press Secretary

NIGER

Head of Delegation

Mr I. B. Mainassara
Minister of Public Health and Social
  Affairs

Delegates

Dr I. M. Djataou
Director of Health Services, Ministry of
  Public Health and Social Affairs

Mr C. K. Hamamane
Chief, Health Education Division

NIGERIA

Head of Delegation

Professor O. Ransome-Kuti
Federal Minister of Health

Delegates

Mr G. Dove-Edwin
High Commissioner of the Federal
  Republic of Nigeria, London

Professor E. M. Essien
Chairman, National Expert Advisory
  Committee on AIDS

Mr F. D. Bolaji
Secretary, National Expert Advisory
  Committee on AIDS

NORWAY

Head of Delegation

Mrs T. S. Gerhardsen*
Minister of Health and Social Affairs

Delegates

Dr S. E. Ekeid
Special Adviser on AIDS Prevention

Mr J. Flatla
Press Counsellor, Royal Norwegian
  Embassy, London

Mrs G. Mollerstad
Personal Adviser to the Minister of
  Health and Social Affairs

Ms I. Ofstand
Royal Norwegian Embassy, London

Mrs A Rikter-Svendsen

Press Attaché, Royal Norwegian
  Embassy, London

Mr K Tonnesen
Consultant

OMAN

Head of Delegation

Dr S. G. H. Al-Akhzami
Under-Secretary, Ministry of Health

Delegates

Dr A. Q. Al-Ghassany
Director of Preventive Medicine,
  Ministry of Health

Mr M. N. Al-Hinai
Health Attaché, Embassy of the
  Sultanate of Oman, London

Dr A. R. Al-Suwaid
Consultant Dermatologist

PANAMA

Head of Delegation

Dr F. Sanchez Cardenas
Minister of Health

Delegates

Mr J. Constantino
Minister Counsellor, Embassy of the
  Republic of Panama, London

Dr. A. Luna
Secretary-General, Ministry of Health

Mr D. Johnson

PAPUA NEW GUINEA

Head of Delegation

Dr T. Ward
Minister of Health

Delegates

Mr R. Kumaina
First Secretary, Ministry of Health

Dr T. Pyakalyia
Assistant Secretary, Disease Control,
  Ministry of Health

PARAGUAY

Head of Delegation

Dr A. Godoy Jimenez
Minister of Public Health and Social
  Welfare

Delegates

Dr A. V. Morales
Director, National Medical Centre

Mr A. R. Zuccolillo
Ambassador of Paraguay, London

POLAND

Head of Delegation

Professor J. Bonczak
Deputy Minister of Health

Delegates

Mrs I. Glowacka
Deputy Director, Department of
  International Relations, Ministry of
  Health and Social Welfare

Professor A. Nowoslawski
Vice-President, AIDS Council

Mr W. Chraniuk
First Secretary, Embassy of the Polish
  People's Republic, London

PORTUGAL

Head of Delegation

Mrs M. L. Beleza
Minister of Health

Delegates

Professor L. Ayres
Head of National AIDS Committee

Dr M. de Lemos
Chief of Cabinet, Ministry of Health

Ms A. Vicente
Health Education Adviser

REPUBLIC OF KOREA

Head of Delegation

Mr Hai-Won Rhee*
Minister of Health and Social Affairs

Delegates

Mr Soon Tae Song

Director, Ministry of Health and Social
  Affairs

Dr Sung Woo Lee
Director-General of Public Health
  Bureau, Ministry of Health and Social
  Affairs

Mr Ui-Guyn Shin
Secretary to the Minister of Health and
  Social Affairs

Mr Tae Kyu Han
Counsellor, Embassy of the Republic of
  Korea, London

ROMANIA

Head of Delegation

Professor V. Ciobanu
Minister of Health

Delegate

Mr D. Tancu
First Secretary, Ministry of Foreign
  Affairs

RWANDA

Head of Delegation

Dr C. Bizimungu
Minister of Public Health and Social
  Affairs

Delegate

Dr D. Nzaramba
Director, Rwandan Campaign against
  AIDS

SAINT LUCIA

Head of Delegation

Mr R. Lansiquot
Minister of Health

Delegate

Mr C. Lubin
Permanent Secretary, Ministry of Health

SAINT VINCENT AND THE
GRENADINES

Head of Delegation

Mr D. Jack
Minister of Health

Delegate
Mr C. F. Browne
Senior Health Educator

SAMOA

Head of Delegation
Mr S. Toeolesulusulu
Minister of Health

Delegate
Dr S. J. Ah-Ching
Chief, Division of Public Health,
　Department of Health

SAN MARINO

Head of Delegation
Dr R. Ghiotti*
Minister of Health and Social Security

Delegate
Dr P. Giacomini
Department of Foreign Affairs

SÃO TOMÉ AND PRINCIPE

Head of Delegation
Mr W. Wilder
Honorary Consul

Delegate
Mrs I. Green

SAUDI ARABIA

Head of Delegation
Mr F. Alhegelan
Minister of Health

Delegates
Dr J. M. Aashy
Assistant Deputy Minister for Preventive
　Medicine, Ministry of Health

Dr I. Al-Sawaygh
General Supervisor for Medical and
　Pharmaceutical Supplies and
　Laboratories

Mr N. H. Qutub
Director, Foreign Relations Department
Ministry of Health

Dr H. K. Khogah
Medical Attaché, Royal Embassy of
　Saudi Arabia, London

SENEGAL

Head of Delegation
Mrs M. Sarr Mbodj
Minister of Health

Delegates
Dr O. Diouf
Chief, National Health Education Unit

Dr I. Ndoye
Co-ordinator and Secretary-General of
　National AIDS Committee

Mr A. F. Faye
First Counsellor, Embassy of the
　Republic of Senegal, London

SEYCHELLES

Head of Delegation
Mr J. Belmont
Minister of Health and Social Services

Delegate
Dr C. Shamlaye
Secretary of State, Ministry of Health
　and Social Services

SIERRA LEONE

Head of Delegation
Dr W. S. B. Johnson*
Minister of Health

Delegates
Dr M. M. Browne
Chief Medical Officer, Ministry of
　Health

Mr S. F. Zack-Williams
Cultural and Information Attaché,
　Sierra Leone High Commission,
　London

SOLOMON ISLANDS

Head of Delegation
Mr J. Tepaika
Minister of Health and Medical Services

Delegates

Dr E. Nukuro
Chief Medical Officer, Ministry of
 Health and Medical Services

Mr M. Tozaka
Permanent Secretary, Ministry of Health
 and Medical Services

SOMALIA

Head of Delegation

Dr M. S. A. Munasar
Minister of Health

Delegate

Dr M. A. Omer
National Programme Manager for
 Sexually Transmitted Diseases

SPAIN

Head of Delegation

Mr J. Garcia Vargas*
Minister of Health and Consumer
 Affairs

Delegates

Dr J. J. Artells
Director-General for Health Planning,
 Ministry of Health and Consumer
 Affairs

Dr A. Infante
Deputy Director-General for
 International Relations, Ministry of
 Health and Consumer Affairs

Miss C. Arredondo
Executive Adviser to the Minister

Dr J. Martinez Salmean
Chief Officer, Severo Ochoa Hospital,
 Madrid

Dr R. de Andres-Medina
Secretary-General for the AIDS
 Problem

Mr L. Fernandez
Private Secretary to the Minister

SRI LANKA

Head of Delegation

Dr R. Atapattu
Minister of Health

Delegates

Dr J. Fernando
Director-General of Health

Mr K. D. Senanayake
Third Secretary, Sri Lanka High
 Commission, London

SUDAN

Head of Delegation

Dr H. S. Abu Salih
Minister of Health and Social Welfare

Delegates

Dr M. Y. Alawad
First Under-Secretary, Ministry of
 Health and Social Welfare

Dr A. Altigani
Director, Virology Department,
 Ministry of Health and Social Welfare

SWAZILAND

Head of Delegation

Dr F. Friedman*
Minister of Health

Delegate

Dr Q. Q. Dlamini
Senior Medical Officer, Ministry of
 Health

SWEDEN

Head of Delegation

Mrs G. Sigurdsen
Minister of Health and Social Affairs

Delegates

Professor L. O. Kallings
Director-General, National
 Bacteriological Laboratory

Mr H. Wrede
Principal Secretary, National
 Commission on AIDS

Dr J. Wallin
Secretary, National Commission on
 AIDS

SWITZERLAND

Head of Delegation
Mr F. Cotti
Federal Councillor; Head, Federal
  Department of the Interior

Delegates
Professor B. A. Roos
Director-General of Public Health,
  Federal Office of Public Health

Dr B. Somaini
Vice-Director, Federal Office of Public
  Health

Dr J. B. Kunz
Counsellor, Swiss Embassy, London

Dr J. Osterwalder
Head, Central AIDS Unit, Federal
  Office of Public Health

THAILAND

Head of Delegation
Mr T. Jayanandana*
Minister of Public Health

Delegates
Dr U. Sudsukh
Director-General, Department of
  Communicable Disease Control,
  Ministry of Public Health

Professor P. Thongcharoen
Head, Department of Microbiology,
  Faculty of Medicine, Mahidol
  University

TOGO

Head of Delegation
Dr A. Dayoka
Director, National Institute of Hygiene

Delegate
Dr A. Edorh
Chief Medical Officer, Department of
  Major Endemic Diseases

TONGA

Head of Delegation
Dr S. Tapa
Minister of Health

Delegate
Mr M. 'Ofanoa
Health Education Officer, Ministry of
  Health

TRINIDAD AND TOBAGO

Head of Delegation
Mr M. O. Assam
High Commissioner for the Republic of
  Trinidad and Tobago, London

Delegates
Mr O. Ali
Deputy High Commissioner, London

Miss R. Ali
First Secretary, Office of the High
  Commissioner for the Republic of
  Trinidad and Tobago, London

TUNISIA

Head of Delegation
Mr H. Khouini*
Ambassador of Tunisia, London

Delegates
Dr M. Sidhom
Director of Preventive Health Care,
  Ministry of Health

Professor R. Gharbi
National AIDS Committee

Mr K. Kaak
Cultural Secretary, Tunisian Embassy,
  London

TURKEY

Head of Delegation
Mr B. Akarcali
Minister of Health and Social Welfare

Delegates
Dr T. Tokgoz
Under-Secretary of State, Ministry of
  Health and Social Welfare

Professor M. Coruh
Member of Supreme Advisory Board on
  AIDS

Dr U. Unsal
Medical Counsellor, Turkish Embassy, London

UGANDA

Head of Delegation
Dr I. J. Batwala*
Deputy Minister of Health

Delegates
Dr S. Etyono
Director of Medical Services, Ministry of Health

Dr I. S. Okware
Chairman, National AIDS Committee

UNION OF SOVIET SOCIALIST REPUBLICS

Head of Delegation
Dr E. I. Chazov
Minister of Health

Delegates
Dr V. P. Sergiev
Chief, Laboratory of Epidemiology and AIDS Prevention

Mr A. M. Vavilov
Counsellor, Ministry of Foreign Affairs

UNITED ARAB EMIRATES

Head of Delegation
Mr H. Al-Madfa
Minister of Health

Delegates
Dr A. W. Al Muhaideb
Assistant Under-Secretary, Ministry of Health

Dr M. Buhannad
Senior Health Administrator, Ministry of Health

Dr Y. M. Al Sadig
Consultant Pathologist

Dr J. Bilal
Medical Attaché, Embassy of the United Arab Emirates, London

UNITED KINGDOM*

Head of Delegation
Mr J. Moore
Secretary of State for Social Services

United Kingdom Ministers
Mrs E. Currie
Parliamentary Under-Secretary of State, Department of Health and Social Security

Mr T. Eggar
Parliamentary Under-Secretary of State, Foreign and Commonwealth Affairs

Mr M. Forsyth
Parliamentary Under-Secretary of State for Scotland

Mr I. Grist
Parliamentary Under-Secretary of State for Wales

Mr R. Needham
Parliamentary Under-Secretary of State for Northern Ireland

Mr T. Newton
Minister for Health, Department of Health and Social Security

Mr M. Rifkind
Secretary of State for Scotland

Lord Skelmersdale
Parliamentary Under-Secretary of State (Lords), Department of Health and Social Security

Department of Health and Social Security
Mr C. W. France
Permanent Secretary

Mr M. Partridge
Second Permanent Secretary

Sir D. Acheson
Chief Medical Officer

Dr E. L. Harris
Deputy Chief Medical Officer

Mr T. S. Heppell
Deputy Secretary

Mrs A. A. B. Poole
Chief Nursing Officer

Ms R. Christopherson
Director, Information

Dr D. Walford
Senior Principal Medical Officer

Mr N. M. Hale
Under-Secretary

Dr H. Pickles
Principal Medical Officer

Mr A. Barton
Assistant Secretary

Dr P. Exon
Senior Medical Officer

Dr G. Greenberg
Senior Medical Officer

Dr H. Williams
Senior Medical Officer

Mr T. Snee
Nursing Officer

Miss D. Dennehy
Nursing Officer

Dr P. A. Hyzler
Senior Medical Officer

Dr G. Lewis
Senior Medical Officer

Dr H. Nicholas
Medical Officer

Mr B. Merkel
Principal

Mr R. Tyrrell
Principal

Mr C. R. Molesworth
Senior Executive Officer

Mr P. McConn
Senior Executive Officer

Scottish Home and Health Department
Dr I. Macdonald
Chief Medical Officer

Mr C. M. A. Lugton
Assistant Secretary

Welsh Office
Mr J. Lloyd
Under-Secretary

*Department of Health and Social
Services, Northern Ireland*
Dr J. McKenna
Chief Medical Officer

Dr R. W. McQuiston
Assistant Secretary

Foreign and Commonwealth Office
Mr J. Poston
Head, Narcotics Control and AIDS
Department

Mr R. Wildash
Desk Officer for AIDS, NCAD

Dr D. Austin
Assistant Desk Officer for AIDS,
NCAD

Overseas Development Administration
Mr J. Caines
Permanent Secretary

Mrs B. Kelly
Head of Health and Population Division

Miss P. Schofield
Senior Executive Officer

Miss M. Pollock
Health Adviser

Miss M. Rutter
Health Adviser

Dr P. Key
Health Adviser

Department of Education and Science
Mrs V. Emmett
Her Majesty's Inspector

Mr B. Peaty
AIDS Unit

Miss C. Bienkowska
AIDS Unit

Mr S. Gane
Science Branch

Mr J. Ungoed Thomas

Department of Employment
Mr G. Kahan

Dependent territories

Anguilla
Mr E. Reid
Minister of Health

Bermuda
Dr J. Cann
Chief Medical Officer

British Virgin Islands
Dr O. Smith
Chief Medical Officer

Falkland Islands
Dr D. Murphy
Chief Medical Officer

Gibraltar
Mr M. K. Featherstone
Minister of Health

Dr A. D. Bacarese-Hamilton
Director of Medical Health

Hong Kong
Mr J. W. Chambers
Secretary for Health and Welfare

Dr E. K. Yeoh
Consultant, Medical and Health
  Department

Mr G. Yuen
Chief Information Officer

Montserrat
Mr V. Jeffers
Minister for Health

Dr L. Lewis
Director of Health Services

Turks and Caicos Islands
Dr H. R. Malcolm
Chief Medical Officer

Crown Dependencies

Isle of Man
Mrs J. Delaney
Junior Minister of Health

Jersey
Deputy M. A. Wavell
Member of Public Health Committee

UNITED REPUBLIC OF TANZANIA

Head of Delegation
Dr A. D. Chiduo*
Minister for Health and Social Welfare

Delegates
Professor S. Y. Maselle
Chairman, National AIDS Task Force

Mrs S. Nyanduga
Third Secretary, High Commission for
  the United Republic of Tanzania,
  London

UNITED STATES OF AMERICA

Head of Delegation
Dr R. E. Windom*
Assistant Secretary for Health

Delegates
Dr C. E. Koop
Surgeon General of the United States

Dr P. J. Fischinger
AIDS Co-ordinator, US Public Health
  Service

Dr G. A. Noble
Deputy Director (AIDS), Centers for
  Disease Control, Atlanta

Dr B. Primm
Presidential AIDS Commission

Dr P. Volberding
Chief, AIDS Programme, San Francisco
  General Hospital

Mr J. Brown
Press Assistant

Dr J. Harris
AIDS Co-ordinator, Agency for
  International Development

URUGUAY

Head of Delegation
Dr R. Ugarte
Minister of Public Health

Delegate
Ms A. Platas
Second Secretary, Embassy of the
  Oriental Republic of Uruguay,
  London

VANUATU

Head of Delegation
Dr O. R. Small
Director of Health; Chairman, AIDS
  Advisory Committee

Delegate
Dr D. Tavoa
Medical Superintendent, Ministry of
  Health

VENEZUELA

Head of Delegation
Mr F. Kerdel-Vegas
Ambassador of Venezuela, London

Delegates
Dr L. A. Blanco Acevedo
Director-General, Health Section,
Ministry of Health and Social Welfare

Mrs Sonia Pittol
Attaché, Venezuelan Embassy, London

VIET NAM

Head of Delegation
Professor Dang Hoi Xuan
Minister of Health

Delegates
Dr Nguyen Van Dong
Director, International Relations
Department, Ministry of Health

Mr Than Nhan Khang
Third Secretary, Embassy of the
Socialist Republic of Viet Nam,
London

YEMEN

Head of Delegation
Dr M. A. Al-Kabab
Minister of Health

Delegates
Dr A. A. Al-Hureibi
Consultant Surgeon, Associate
Professor, Sana'a University

Dr A. A. Wali Nasher
Associate Professor of Surgery, Sana'a
University

Mr K. Al-Sakkaf
Director, International Health
Relations, Ministry of Health

YUGOSLAVIA

Head of Delegation
Dr J. Obocki
President, Federal Committee for
Labour, Health and Social Welfare

Delegates
Dr N. Georgievski
Assistant to the President, Federal
Committee for Labour, Health and
Social Welfare

Dr S. Lang
President, Health and Social Council,
Zagreb

ZAIRE

Head of Delegation
Dr B. N'Galy
Director, AIDS Control Programme

Delegates
Dr B. Likinda
Medical Adviser

Ms Omba Mafama Ngandu
Director, Paediatrics Department,
University Clinic, Kinshasa

ZAMBIA

Head of Delegation
Mr R. C. Sakuhuka
Minister of Health

Delegates
Mr S. Mutondo
Acting High Commissioner for the
Republic of Zambia, London

Dr S. L. Nyaywa
Assistant Director of Medical Services,
Ministry of Health

Mr O. C. Lungwe
Second Secretary, High Commission for
the Republic of Zambia, London

ZIMBABWE

Head of Delegation
Mr F. Muchemwa
Minister of Health

Delegates
Dr H. M. Murerwa
High Commissioner for the Republic of
Zimbabwe, London

Dr D. G. Makuto
Permanent Secretary, Ministry of Health

Dr J. C. Emmanuel
Medical Director, Blood Transfusion
  Service

Dr B. Manyame
National Maternal and Child Health Co-
  ordinator

**REPRESENTATIVE OF THE WHO
EXECUTIVE BOARD**

Dr A. Grech
Chairman

**REPRESENTATIVES OF THE UNITED
NATIONS AND RELATED
ORGANIZATIONS**

United Nations
Mr R. Ahmed
Under-Secretary General

Miss M. Anstee
Director-General, United Nations Office
  at Vienna

Mrs M. Kennedy
Information Officer

*United Nations Children's Fund
  (UNICEF)*
Ms E. A. Preble
Senior Project Officer, AIDS
  Programme

*United Nations Development Programme
  (UNDP)**
Mr A. Ajello
Assistant Administrator

*United Nations Population Fund
  (UNFPA)*
Dr J. Donayre
Acting Chief, Technical and Evaluation
  Division

*International Narcotics Control Board
  (INCB)*
Mr S. R. Ali Khan
President

International Labour Office
Mr J. de Martino
Mr D. Richardson
Office for International Relations

*United Nations Educational, Scientific
  and Cultural Organization
  (UNESCO)**
Mr B Biyong
Chief, Education for Quality of Life
  Section

World Bank
Mrs A. Hamilton
Director, Population and Human
  Resources Department

Dr A. Measham
Health Adviser

**REPRESENTATIVES OF OTHER
INTERGOVERNMENTAL
ORGANIZATIONS**

African Development Bank
Dr R. Wanji Ngah
Senior Health Expert

Council of Europe
Mr J. F. Smyth*
Director of Social and Economic Affairs

*Council Secretariat of the European
  Communities*
Mr W. Gaede
Principal Administrator

*Commission of the European
  Communities*
Dr A. Baert
Director-General

Commonwealth Secretariat
Professor K. Thairu
Medical Adviser

Dr K. W. Edmondson
Assistant Director

Inter-American Development Bank
Mr H. E. Luisi
United Kingdom Representative

League of Arab States
Mr M. Mustafa Al-Hadi
Assistant Secretary-General

Dr B. Samara
Specialist

Organization of African Unity
Dr A. Salama
Head, Health Bureau

Organization of Economic Co-operation and Development
Dr C. Wahren
Head, AIDS Management Division

REPRESENTATIVES OF NONGOVERNMENTAL ORGANIZATIONS IN OFFICIAL RELATIONS WITH WHO

Christian Medical Commission
Mrs B. Rubenson
Programme Secretary

International Council of Nurses
Mr T. Clay
Member, Board of Directors

International Council on Alcohol and Addictions
Dr S. Malik
Director of Research

International League against the Venereal Diseases and the Treponematoses
Dr A. Siboulet
President

Dr M. A. Waugh
General Secretary

International Planned Parenthood Federation
Dr P. Senanayake
Assistant Secretary-General

Dr A. Klouda
Co-ordinator, AIDS Unit

International Society of Blood Transfusion
Dr W. Wagstaff
Director, Regional Transfusion Centre, Sheffield, United Kingdom

International Union for Health Education
Dr H. Crawley
President

Dr M. F. Silverman
President, American Foundation for AIDS Research

League of Red Cross and Red Crescent Societies
Dr B. Dick
Head, Community Health Department

Save the Children Fund
Mr N. Hinton
Director-General

Dr P. Poore
Medical Officer

World Federation of Hemophilia
Mr D. Watters
General Secretary, United Kingdom

World Federation for Medical Education
Professor H. J. Walton
President

REPRESENTATIVES OF OTHER INVITED ORGANIZATIONS

Association of Directors of Social Services
Ms D. Platt

Association of Directors of Social Work (Lothian Region)
Mr R. W. Kent

British Association for Counselling
Mr A. Grey

British Association of Social Workers
Mr R. Gaitley

British Medical Association
Professor M. Adler

British Psychological Society
Mr A. Bucknall

British Pharmacological Society
Dr J. K. Aronson

The Conference of the Royal Colleges of the United Kingdom
Dame Barbara Clayton
Dr E. R. Rue

General Visitors' Association
Mrs A. Game

Institute of Environmental Health Officers
Mr I. S. Gray

Royal College of Midwives
Miss G. Balfour

Royal College of Nursing
Mr R. J. Wells

*United Kingdom Central Council of
   Nurses, Midwives and Health Visitors*
Mr R. H. Pyne

Medical Research Council
Dr D. A. Rees

AIDS Consortium for the Third World
Ms M. Haslegrave
Ms Hughes
Dr C. Moreno

AIDS Helpline (Northern Ireland)
Miss J. Macrae

AIDS Network SCOAN
Mr D. Critchard
Mr R. Goodwin
Mr T. Hurn
Mr D. Langley
Ms J. Springham

Body Positive
Mr D. Hudson

Family Planning Association
Mr P. Gordon
Ms Z. Pauncefort
Mr A. Service

The Haemophilia Society
Rev. A. J. Tanner

Health Education Authority
Sir Brian Bailey
Dr S. Hagard
Ms S. Perl

National AIDS Trust
Ms J. McKessack

*National Council for Voluntary
   Organisations*
Mr S. Hebditch

Scottish AIDS Monitor
Mr B. Devlin

*Scottish Health Education Group
   (SHEG)*
Mr S. Mitchell
Mr M. J. Raymond

*Standing Conference on Drug Abuse
   (SCODA)*
Mr D. Turner

The Terrence Higgins Trust
Mr J. Fitzpatrick

Welsh Health Promotion Authority
Dr S. A. Smail

UNITED KINGDOM OBSERVERS

Mr M. R. Bailey
London School of Hygiene and Tropical
   Medicine

Professor R. Cawley
Institute of Psychiatry, London

Professor R. Frankenberg
Social Anthropology and Social Work
   Centre for Medical Social
   Anthropology, London

Dr P. P. Mortimer
Public Health Laboratory Service

Dr D. N. Nabarro
Liverpool School of Tropical Medicine

Dr A. J. Pinching
Saint Mary's Medical School, London

Mr R. J. Pratt
Charing Cross School of Nursing

Sir John Reid
Consultant Adviser to the Chief Medical
   Officer on International Health

Dr C. E. G. Smith
Dean, London School of Hygiene and
   Tropical Medicine

Dr R. Tedder
Head of Virology
The Middlesex Hospital, London

Professor S. Wallman
University College Hospital, London

Professor A. J. Zuckerman
Director, Department of Microbiology,
   London School of Hygiene and
   Tropical Medicine

Steering Committee

Co-chairmen

Sir Donald Acheson, Chief Medical Officer, Department of Health and Social Security, United Kingdom

Dr J. Mann, Director, Global Programme on AIDS, World Health Organization, Geneva, Switzerland

Members

Mr N. Hale, Department of Health and Social Security, United Kingdom

Mr G. Lupton, Department of Health and Social Security, United Kingdom

Dr P. Mason, Department of Health and Social Security, United Kingdom

Co-secretaries

Ms K. Kay, Global Programme on AIDS, Geneva, Switzerland
Mrs J. Mixer, Department of Health and Social Security, United Kingdom

Secretariat

WORLD HEALTH ORGANIZATION OFFICIALS

Dr H. Mahler
Director-General

Dr H. A. Gezairy
Regional Director for the Eastern Mediterranean

Dr J. E. Asvall
Regional Director for Europe

Dr U. Ko Ko
Regional Director for South-East Asia

Dr H. Nakajima
Regional Director for the Western Pacific

Dr J. Cohen
Adviser on Health Policy

Mrs I. Brüggemann
Director, Programme for External Coordination

Mrs A. Kern
Director, Division of Public Information and Education for Health

Dr G. Mutalik
Director, Liaison Office with the United Nations, New York

Mr C. H. Vignes
Legal Counsel

Dr E. G. Beausoleil
Chairman, AIDS Task Force, Regional Office for Africa

Mr T. B. Ndiaye
Chief, Public Information and Education for Health, Regional Office for Africa

Dr N. Drager
External Relations Officer

Mrs K. Metwalli
Conference Officer

Mrs A. M. Mutschler
Protocol Officer

WHO GLOBAL PROGRAMME ON AIDS

Dr J. Mann
Director

Mr J. Bunn
Public Information Officer

Dr M. Carballo
Chief, Social and Behavioural Research Unit

Dr J. Chin
Chief, Surveillance Forecasting and Impact Assessment Unit

Dr J. Esparza
Acting Chief, Biomedical Research Unit

Ms S. Gianou
Consultant, National Programme Support Unit

Sir James Gowans
Consultant, Biomedical Research Unit

Ms K. Kay
Office of the Director

Dr A. Meyer
Chief, Health Promotion Unit

Mr T. Mooney
External Relations Officer

Mr T. Netter
Public Information Officer

Dr G. Slutkin
Consultant

Dr D. Tarantola
Chief, National Programme Support Unit

Mr J. Wickett
Consultant

Dr R. Widdus
Chief, Programme Coordination and Development

Secretariat

Miss D. Appiah
Mrs E. Bernard
Miss A. F. Canaud
Miss C. Hanganaqui
Miss C. Greasley
Mrs L. Hediger

Miss R. Kissenberger
Mrs P. Leccia
Miss P. Ratcliffe
Miss C. Rose
Mrs J. Wylie

UNITED KINGDOM

Department of Health and Social Security

Sir Donald Acheson
Chief Medical Officer

Mr N. M. Hale
Under-Secretary

Mr G. C. M. Lupton
Assistant Secretary

Dr P. Mason
Senior Medical Officer

Summit Administrative Liaison Team

Mrs J. Mixer
Ms M. Kirk
Ms J. Wood
Miss J. Doolan

Information Division

Mr P. Wilson
Deputy Director

Mr G. Meredith
Deputy Director

Mr M. Reid
Principal Information Officer

Ms C. Murphy
Senior Information Officer

Mr S. Bird
Higher Executive Officer

Index

Cayman Islands, AIDS cases 126
Central African Republic, AIDS
    cases 125
Chad, AIDS cases 125
Child Survival Initiatives 7
children with AIDS 23, 108–10
Chile, AIDS cases 126
China (Province of Taiwan), AIDS
    cases 128
church, role in education 34
Colombia, AIDS cases 126
condoms 10, 11, 15, 18, 19, 31, 38, 39,
    42, 52, 53, 55, 56, 57, 60–61, 63,
    67, 68, 69–71, 89
Congo, AIDS cases 125
Costa Rica, AIDS cases 126
Côte d'Ivoire, AIDS cases 126
Council of Europe 65
counselling 10, 11, 53, 67, 75–94, 120,
    123, 132
    after HIV testing 86–9
    before HIV testing 82–5
    persons with AIDS 90–4
Cuba, AIDS cases 126
Cyprus, AIDS cases 128
Czechoslovakia, AIDS cases 127

Denmark,
    AIDS cases 127
    focus on adolescents 54–8
discrimination 10–11, 56, 91, 105, 123,
    132
disinformation 36
Dominica, AIDS cases 126
Dominican Republic, AIDS cases 126
drug abusers, HIV transmission 16 (see
    also intravenous drug users)

Ebola fever 17
Ecuador, AIDS cases 126
Egypt, AIDS cases 128
El Salvador, AIDS cases 126
ethical considerations 19, 64, 104
Ethiopia, AIDS cases 125
Europe,
    AIDS cases 4, 129, 130
    AIDS epidemiology 5, 6
European Economic Community 65

family counselling 88–9, 93
Finland, AIDS cases 127

Folio 26
France,
    AIDS cases 28, 127
    National AIDS Information
        Programme 28–31
French Guiana, AIDS cases 126
French Polynesia, AIDS cases 128

Gabon, AIDS cases 125
Gambia, AIDS cases 125
genital ulcer 15
German Democratic Republic, AIDS
    cases 127
Germany, Federal Republic of, AIDS
    cases 127
Ghana, AIDS cases 125
Greece, AIDS cases 127
Grenada, AIDS cases 126
Guadeloupe, AIDS cases 126
Guatemala, AIDS cases 126
Guinea, AIDS cases 125
Guinea-Bissau, AIDS cases 125
Guyana, AIDS cases 126

haemophilia 17
Haiti, AIDS cases 126
health care system 105
"health promotion" 24–7, 72–3, 120
health workers xxi, 9, 10
    education/training 30, 37–8, 95,
        97–100, 102, 120
    infection from patients 17
    psychological stress 101, 103–7,
        108–9
    role in public education 59–61, 110
    support 95, 100–102, 103
hepatitis B 17, 64, 100
heterosexual transmission 5, 6, 15, 23,
    42, 52–3
homosexual men 5, 12, 38, 39, 42–3,
    51, 64, 69–71, 87, 88, 104
homosexual transmission 5, 6, 15, 41
Honduras, AIDS cases 126
Hong Kong, AIDS cases 128
Hot Rubber Company 70–71
human immunodeficiency virus
    (HIV) 3
    infection rates 3–4
    modes of transmission xvii, 4, 5,
        15–18, 25, 33, 131–2
    screening/testing 11, 30, 31, 53,
        82–4, 100, 104, 109, 132, 133–4